Magic for Longevity

How I Stay Fit, Healthy and Happy

By

Antonina Duridanova

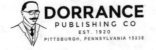

DORRANCE
PUBLISHING CO
EST. 1920
PITTSBURGH, PENNSYLVANIA 15238

Dorrance Publishing Co
585 Alpha Drive
Suite 103
Pittsburgh, PA 15238
Visit our website at *www.dorrancebookstore.com*

ISBN: 979-8-88925-205-4
eISBN: 979-8-88925-705-9

Contents

Magic for Longevity: How I Stay Fit, Healthy and Happy

Introduction

I am seventy-three years old, and a mother of three children, but people think that I am twenty years younger. I am not taking any medicine and rarely use supplements. "What do you do to look so youthful?" A question I hear all the time. A mother wished her daughter for her birthday to look as good as me when she is seventy. When I gave my date of birth to a guy in Cancun filling out a form to get a kayak, he thought that I made a mistake in saying 1949; he thought I meant 1969. "My mother looks nothing like you, and she is your age. What is your secret for looking and acting so youthfully?" I heard such comments more than once from younger women and men.

All the compliments and questions about my appearance prompted me to write this book about aspects of my life that have brought me joy and kept me mentally, physically, and spiritually fit. I hope my readers find this information interesting and helpful.

To what people see as my youthful appearance, I need to add that I am grateful to have the energy to engage in the activities that I currently enjoy—yoga, walking, hiking, biking, swimming, dancing, snorkeling, and traveling.

It is also important to have a sound mind. I published a book in English and Bulgarian languages. Promoting the book takes me to different states and cities, giving presentations, having book signings, meeting wonderful people, and making new friendships. I also take piano lessons and study Chinese. I enjoyed painting as a child, so I started to paint, and any chance I have I visit art galleries and museums.

I know if I ask you "Do you want to live up to a hundred years while being mobile and with all your mental capacities?" the answer will be: "You bet." So how can we manage to have a long, productive, happy life? Is there a formula on how to preserve our looks and vitality? In today's world of technology, we are bombarded with all kinds of miracle pills, claiming to slow the process of aging. And then we have all recipes on what and how to exercise usually cited in an order of one to ten or twenty, and people are frantically trying to apply them in their short, busy days. Some folks set an alarm as a reminder to do sit ups, push-ups, or start on a ten-thousand-step walking routine.

My friendly doctors will respond that longevity is due to genes, and I do not dispute that theory. However, we as individuals have the power to change the way we look and feel. We can adopt new ways and styles of living, which include our views on life, our nourishment, exercising, approach to problem solving, we can expand our horizons by visiting new places and learning about other people's customs and habits.

The following sections reveal what I do in terms of exercise, nutrition, weight control, mental and spiritual well-being, and the pleasures I derive from visiting art museums and traveling the world.

In my opinion, which is based on my experiences, travel is the most significant activity for energizing simultaneously the body and spirit. It provides exclusive benefits, ranging from improved cardiovascular system to memory enhancement. Therefore, you will find most of my book describing touring amazing countries in Africa, Asia, South America, and Europe, which is considered the cradle of Western civilization.

Reading chapters of the book, you will learn about the diverse activities that I enjoy and that are close to my heart, which I perform in moderation, without rigid schedules or following routines. You will find out that I customize my daily workout schedule to take pleasure in the exercises and/or activities that I choose. Medical science tells us that such an approach in exercising releases dopamine in our bodies, a chemical known to boost the mood.

In conclusion I would like to say that this is not a textbook. I am not a nutritionist or expert in the health field. This book is designed to share my personal experiences and knowledge in keeping a healthy body, mind, and soul. I hope that you find my discussions helpful to improve the quality of your life.

CHAPTER 1
Physical And Mental Fitness—
Food for the Body and Mind

I believe that exercise and proper nutrition are the keys to staying fit. I have been fortunate to learn to be physically active from early childhood, so what I do to stay fit comes naturally from habit and not from routines suggested by others. And I grew up on a healthy diet provided by my grandmother. Subsequently I developed my love for exercise and proper nutrition that has kept me physically fit throughout the years. I have also adopted a lifestyle which allows me to pursue my interests and has contributed to my mental and spiritual fitness. Those activities include hobbies, travel, relationships, meditation, and stress-reduction techniques in handling demanding situations as COVID and life transitions. I constantly engage in learning new skills, subjects, materials, and topics that I am interested in such as music, art, and travel.

I have loved reading, writing, music, drawing, painting, travel, yoga, swimming, hiking, biking, and much more for as long as I remember. The effect of engaging in all these activities is tremendous as they interact with each other and when practiced with pleasure, make us feel happy, which is reflected in our appearance. I do not follow a specific daily schedule. While it is important to plan, I do it in a loose, unstructured way. I might play the piano early in the morning or late at night, and same with writing, reading, or painting, which I alternate with physical exercises.

Before I retired, I had a very demanding job. I also raised three children and took care of my mother. Regardless of my busy schedule I managed to live a healthy lifestyle by balancing work and home with activities that I enjoyed from an early age, as well as adding new ones. When I had a family with children at home, we spent a lot of our time outdoors, and I always planned trips by water or the hillside.

The following sections describe activities that have sustained me physically and mentally fit through good and troublesome times.

EXERCISE

I have kept fit by performing various activities, not all of them daily and not at a set time. I do not follow a strict routine, and I do not keep a list of things to do in a race to be healthy. Instead, I choose my activities every day, based on my mood and what my body prompts me to do. For example, as I wake up, stretching in bed and having my first coffee, I might feel like it is a day for biking, swimming, dancing, and I will squeeze in a short routine of yoga to keep my body flexible. I like the Indian yoga instructors on YouTube. They give me the necessary workout and make me smile during their sessions.

Medical science informs us that the uplifted mood we get from exercise is because of endorphins in the body that interact with receptors from the brain, and the result is best when we perform activities that we love. Walking ten thousand steps sounds to me like an obligation and even punishment. I walk because I like to be outdoors where I admire nature, listening to the birds' chirping and feeling the wind caressing my face. And when in town I like looking at the crowds passing by, the store windows of clothes and food, and the people sitting at outdoor cafes and restaurants.

What I observe is that folks tend to rely on methods prescribed by others and apply them unwillingly such as using the stairs instead of taking the elevator. So, what if you are coming from a swim or working out at the gym? Do you really need to puff up the stairs? I try not to overexert my body doing something I don't like. Physical activities need to be pleasurable, and there are so many to choose from: fishing and playing golf will relax your mind; surfing, boat rowing and sailing will raise your adrenaline; and the list goes on. In cold weather there is sledding, skating, skiing, walking, and much more. I do not like the cold, but I like the outdoors, so when I lived in Michigan, instead of staying in, I went sledding with the kids, made snowmen, and took walks by Lake Huron. As a teenager in Bulgaria, I even started to ski when I was seventeen. I will never forget my first downhill experience on a small mountain Lyulin by Sofia—my native city. I don't know how many times I fell, but I figured out how to take the turns and arrived all happy and vigorous at the foot of the mountain.

We are usually advised that when it comes to physical fitness, we need to move, otherwise we will get very sick, and I believe that this statement is not far from the truth. I am not an avid sports person, but I learned to love the outdoor activities as a child on the slopes of the hills and the meadows at my grandmother's village near Rakelovtsi. I also played outside any chance I got in my hometown Sofia, a city at the foot of the Vitosha Mountain, where on weekends residents hiked and had picnics.

Growing up in the city I could play dodgeball, hide and seek, and tag in the street in front of our apartment building, and I spent my summers at my grandmother's village roaming the hills and valleys barefoot until dusk. Hopping on the back of a horse with my cousin, exploring the countryside and visiting villagers in houses scattered on the hills with old walnut trees in their yards gave me tremendous pleasure. In the evening we would get back to the old house built with wooden walls filled with mud and straw, and a hearth in the front room where the women cooked the meals.

Those were happy days as I recall every morning running out with bread and cheese in my hand, feeling the grass on my feet, the breeze in my face, and the sunlight warming my body. I smelled the scents of the wildflowers, admired the sight of ravines and mountaintops, and the sound of birds and felt just wonderful. From there on I took any opportunity I had to be outdoors and hiked, swam, played tennis, volleyball, basketball, and even golf once on vacation with my younger daughter.

Later in my adult life, with a demanding job and family, I managed to squeeze in time to work out at the gym, picking up exercises I liked—swimming, yoga, aerobics, and dance. On weekends we went hiking, bike riding, visiting festivals and art galleries, and attending concerts, the latter became more possible in Texas, as I started to engage in more cultural activities which I missed from my childhood.

Following is a list of physical activities that I enjoy and practice:

a. Swimming – I live in Texas, and I enjoy swimming at the community pool twice or three times a week. I usually do twelve to fourteen laps at my own pace, choosing any style that keeps me moving. This exercise gives me a great deal of energy, since movement in the water and under the sun is both physically and spiritually stimulating. I cannot describe the euphoria I feel when I dip myself in the water and float or dive under. My aunt introduced me to this miracle exercise when she took me on vacation to the Black Sea and taught me how to swim, for which I am extremely grateful. I was eight or nine when I discovered how moving up and down with the waves and floating on my back, letting them carry me to the shore, was such a thrill. It is no wonder that swimming, apart from being a physical exercise, brings happiness, because it causes the release of endorphins in our brain—a chemical producing a good sensation, lowering stress, increasing pleasure, and reducing pain. Physical therapists prescribe swimming as effective and manageable exercise for accident victims, and I believe it can also be used to improve mental health.

b. Snorkeling – Snorkeling is even more enjoyable, as the feeling of swimming with fish and turtles over beautiful corals is exuberating. I was taught when swimming to keep my head above the water, so it took me some time to feel comfortable dipping myself under water, but once I did it, a new world of beauty opened in front of my eyes. I started to snorkel when I was sixty-four while on a cruise in the Pacific Ocean. We were on a private island when Mitt gave me the snorkels and swam away. I did not know how to properly use them, so I kept gagging trying to put them on. I was so happy when a woman snorkeling close by came over to help me. Since then, I tried snorkeling on different trips, some in the Caribbean and the Maldives, but water kept coming both in the mask and the snorkel, so I had to adjust them constantly. Nonetheless I was getting the thrill of snorkeling for the brief times that I was underwater. Then it dawned on me to visit a specialty store for snorkeling and diving equipment, and that changed my entire experience. I was so happy to be able to stay longer underwater, swim farther, and encounter more beautiful fish of different colors and shapes. Since I learned how to snorkel, whenever I put on a mask and fins and dive in, I feel a rush of excitement and joy from the thrill of being in the marine world. I must admit that I am not brave about swimming with stingrays, snakes, and sharks. I had a close encounter a couple of times with sting rays which terrified me. One time I was bold and decided to swim from the corals to the very dark-blue-colored water, where it was extremely deep. Suddenly I noticed the black shape of a stingray shooting up rather fast from the bottom to the surface towards me. I gathered all my strength and swam as fast as I could to get away. This happened by Bora Bora Island, where the waters are full of sharks and stingrays, and I swear that people feed them before taking tourists on private boat trips to swim with them. Another time we were at Amedee Island in New Caledonia, which is known for the abundance of sea turtles swimming up to the shore. I am always cautious when in unknown waters, so I decided to snorkel off the beach without going too far out. And then I saw it, a big, beautiful turtle. My heart was pounding as I started to swim parallel to it when, suddenly, I noticed a snake on the other side of the turtle. That ended my snorkeling for the day, but I had a story to tell and felt so happy that I could swim alongside a turtle. Why was I feeling so exuberant and full of joy when snorkeling? As in swimming, the release of endorphins in the brain causes this high-spirited ecstatic feeling of pleasure, serving as mood enhancer and stress relief. What are the benefits of snorkeling? Swimming longer underwater requires physical exertion, which results in improved cardiovascular health, added to joint and muscle strengthening. And let's not forget the burning of calories and toning up. In my case I could also feel the adrenaline flowing through my veins as I was floating over corals and spotting fish.

c. Kayaking is another outdoor, very pleasurable sport, as every stroke you make with the oars fills your lungs with fresh air, increases your strength, and enhances your mood. My first kayaking was at a man-made small lake in Sofia by the Tsar Boris Park. My cousins who lived in the same apartment building, and whose parents were instructors in physical education, suggested that we go to the lake and rent a boat. The couple of hours we spent rowing the boat were a new thrilling experience for me. I felt happy feeling the wind in my face as we maneuvered the boat.

Rowing is an exercise that involves a full workout of your body muscles; it is more pleasing when done outdoors, rather than with rowing equipment at home or at the gym. I remember spending hours kayaking with my daughter when we were on vacation in Cozumel. It was not only useful physical exercise, but it was also extremely pleasant. First, it was enjoyable to be with my daughter, and then there were the added factors of enjoyment from exercising at sea. As in snorkeling, I get excited when kayaking, and my heart starts beating a little faster at the prospect of discovering the direction of the tide and how far out to go.

I remember another occasion kayaking in Cancun. It was a white sandy beach with enticing blue waters. Sitting under the umbrella I had the urge to try kayaking, so, armed with oars, I hopped on the boat and took off, as happy as I could be. My enjoyment increased with every stroke, making me feel more confident and braver. The known chemicals which were producing this effect on me were the neurotransmitters serotonin, dopamine, and endorphins. The list of benefits from kayaking is long—it tones the legs, arms, and core; it increases endurance; it contributes to better focus; it also reduces stress and helps with sleeping.

d. Walking – I like to walk, and when I worked, I felt jealous of people in the neighborhood who had the luxury to stroll whenever they felt like it. I still walked after work, if I did not have time to go to the gym. Now that I am retired, I can walk whenever I like, preferably in the morning before engaging in my intellectual and social activities for the day, but I also walk in the evening. I do not walk too fast, always choosing a pace that suits my mood and my body. This is important to me because I like to keep a balance between my physical and mental state. Somebody has come up with a theory that we all need to walk ten thousand steps a day to be healthy, and Mitt, my husband, gave me a watch to count my steps, which is something that many people are suddenly doing. What I discovered is that my body dictates the number of steps I need to take, especially if I do other physical exercises. Sometimes I can walk for an hour, which gets me the ten thousand steps, other times I am in the mood to do less. What matters is how I feel at the end of the day—energetic and content, or sluggish, which prompts me to adjust my next day's routine. But as a rule, I exercise daily for a couple of hours.

e. Hiking – Like running, hiking can appear undesirable and strenuous, but hiking is more than just an exercise; it also allows you to be in touch with nature and admire your surroundings. The feeling is immense, as you fill your lungs with clean air and feel more energetic; your heart starts to beat faster, and once on top of the hill your chest expands and the blood rushes through your body. When I was

7

young, I used to hike regularly on Vitosha Mountain, but when I returned to Bulgaria after living in Michigan for years, I discovered that I could not go too far up the mountain. Starting at the very bottom from a place called Dragalevtsi, I puffed up for about an hour and then decided that I needed to reward myself at the nearby restaurant with a glass of Bulgarian Zagorka beer and a meal of *kebapche*—a Bulgarian very tasty kebab. The following week I went higher up to the first stop of the lift and rewarded myself again. I continued with this routine until I reached Lodge Aleko 1,810 m. above sea level. From there on the hike was pleasant as the terrain changed to a plateau—a relatively flat terrain almost bare, which goes across to the other end of the mountain. At that point I took a bus down to the city. When I returned to Sofia, I tried to find my old acquaintances and came upon a young woman who was one of my mother's former students. She was also a mountaineer and we started to hike every Sunday for about seven hours regardless of the weather starting at Vladaya, crossing the plateau to Lodge Aleko and walking down to Bai Krastjo—a stop of the chairlift. Here I had again my meal of kebapche, with tea and cognac. From there we took the lift down to the city, energized to start a new work week. I need to mention that we were not racing up the mountain; we took our time, stopping to rejoice in the scenery and admire nature in the summer and winter seasons. Our Sunday hiking kept me energized until Thursday, when I looked forward to the weekend to do it over again. At work I felt happy, more concentrated, and productive, completing my tasks with ease.

Now I live in San Antonio, Texas, and there are no big mountains to conquer here, but the city is in the hill country, and there are parks where you can hike—Eisenhower, Friedrichs Park, etc., so any chance Mitt and I get, we climb the hills of these parks for a couple of hours and sometimes for as much as four hours.

What is the reason for the elevation of spirits, clarity, and effectiveness at work after hiking? When climbing up a mountain and reaching a peak, or the top of a hill, there is a rush of adrenaline in your body which triggers an increase of dopamine in the brain—a hormone referred to as a happy hormone, and happy people are more productive. Hiking helps combat depression and anxiety as nature heals the soul, offering scenes of beautiful streams running down a hill, of colorful wildflowers, bushes with wild berries, and majestic evergreen trees with pinecones on the ground that you can take home for souvenirs. These are times when you forget problems, absorbed in the scenery around you, feeling overcome by peace and tranquility.

   f. Biking – I started biking at the age of forty-three when I was on assignment in Bulgaria as US tax advisor. My daughters, who were eleven and twenty-two, liked to bike in the city of Sofia. It got them around faster, and they enjoyed the exercise. So, I started to bike with them. I bought myself a bike and slowly made progress, learning how to maneuver among the crowds in the streets. It was on the first days of biking when I discovered that unlike skiing, you do not stop by lowering your body to the side. It was a painful learning experience when I fell and scraped my knees. I walked my bike home, washed up, and decided that since I liked my new exercise, I had to learn how to do it properly. I gradually increased the distance that I biked and started to enjoy not just the exercise but also the feeling it was giving me of freedom and happiness. Somehow the anxiety or worries of the day dissipated when I rode the bike after work from our apartment in downtown Sofia to the foot of the mountain in Knyazhevo.

When I returned to Texas, I wanted to resume bike riding, but it seemed difficult at first as I felt wobbly and unstable. After struggling on my own for a while I remembered a woman at work who was bike riding with a group, and I decided to join them. I felt anxious, as I was driving to the meeting place downtown San Antonio. But everybody seemed very nice, and I felt reassured when I heard that they never leave anybody behind. I was very apprehensive of every move I made, but I was rolling along with everybody else. The one difficulty I had was starting again when we had to stop at traffic lights, but I kept up without being unsure or wobbly. I found out that following the person in front of me made me feel confident. The group had a routine that called for riding and stopping halfway for breakfast at one of the mom-and-pop taco restaurants, and I remember how on my first day I arrived at one of these places soaking wet. That day I rode twenty miles with everybody else. I joined the group one more time and feeling already confident to ride on my own, I stopped going with them as I did not want to slow everybody down. But their influence on me was tremendous, and even now when I go up a hill, I can hear the voice of my fellow riders encouraging me to just pedal. And I fulfilled my wish to bike the Missions in San Antonio, joining in a scheduled event to celebrate the city's anniversary. I joined a group biking ten miles and had one of the most pleasant experiences, as we stopped to visit the different missions and enjoyed the park surroundings. Now biking is one of my weekly exercises which I alternate with other activities—swimming, hiking, yoga. The benefits I receive from biking are numerous. It increases muscle strength and flexibility, and I feel strong and energetic; it improves my posture and coordination, it decreases fat levels in my body (proven by annual medical checkups), it alleviates any stress I might experience, and strengthens my bones and my cardiovascular fitness. And since I mentioned how biking made me happy, one can guess that it is due to the release of serotonin and dopamine, the chemicals in the bloodstream causing euphoria and pain relief. Serotonin is the chemical responsible for your positive feelings and self-confidence found in exercises I already described above such as kayaking and snorkeling. Some people use stationary bikes, but the benefit is far greater if you are outdoors absorbing vitamin D and admiring nature and outdoor life.

    g. Yoga – My yoga experience started in Dallas. One day a colleague from work mentioned that she was going to the Federal Employees gym during lunch, and I decided to join her. The building was only a couple of blocks away, and as I entered, I spotted the weight machines and equipment on the right side. On the left was an exercise room, and people were sitting on their mats, waiting for the start of a yoga class. I grabbed a mat, too, and was happy to find a spot in the front. Soon the instructor walked in, a young, tall, well-built African American with a friendly smile. The session lasted an hour, and I did everything possible to follow the poses, appreciating at the end the *shavasana*, feeling my body relaxing and my mind being calm. I was surprised that when I returned to the office and sat at the desk my hips were not aching; I felt refreshed and better focused on the afternoon work. From that day on I never missed that guy's sessions. I will always remember him saying: "If you do not do yoga, you will not be able to bend down and tie your shoes when you are sixty." I was fifty-four at the time, and I believed him as I felt such a relief after only a one-hour yoga on the first day. When I moved to Houston and later San Antonio, I continued practicing group yoga at LA Fitness and Golds gym, which I visited twice a week after work. I loved the benefits from yoga. It made me feel stronger, toned up, more flexible, and relaxed. When all gyms closed after COVID, I found yoga instructors on YouTube and picked up an Indian instructor who had diverse programs, including ones that invigorate and strengthen the body and others for stretching and falling sleep. These practices are from ten to thirty minutes and can be combined to achieve different results. If I run late, I will do at least fifteen minutes of stretching. I started to do the exercises outside on the patio, which makes the experience far more enjoyable because I can look at the grass, bushes, trees, flowers, and can listen to the birds singing while doing the poses. I am convinced that yoga is a practice for the body, soul, and mind because of the results I derive from it. It is the best conditioning exercise because it tones up the muscles without the use of heavy weights. Balancing poses not only strengthen the muscles, but they also calm the mind.

I remember how after stressful days at work, yoga made me feel relieved and uplifted my mood.

Yoga has become a part of my daily routine and I cannot imagine life without it. I do not look for creams and pills when my neck, shoulders, or hips are stiff or when I have a headache. There are yoga poses that alleviate all kinds of aches and pains, so yoga is what I do when I feel any discomfort.

Following are some helpful basic yoga poses:
1. Cat Cow position strengthens and stretches the spine, the hips, the back, and it also reduces stress.
2. A Downward-Facing Dog Pose strengthens the hands, wrists, arms, and shoulders as well as the calves and hamstrings; it lengthens the spine, it clears up sinuses, increases blood flow to the brain, and calms the nerves.
3. Bridge Pose tones the muscles and the core as well as stretches the legs and back. Performing it with control is known to reduce anxiety.
4. Plank Pose is recommended for good posture, strengthening of the spine and the core muscles, the rhomboids and trapezius. It is also used for weight control because it increases metabolism. Plank Pose is known to attack knots and strain muscles which in turn reduces anxiety and stress.
5. Child's Pose offers good stretching, calms the nervous system, soothes the mind, and restores peace to the soul. It is one of my favorite poses after strenuous mental or physical work.

All yoga poses align the body and the mind to function simultaneously, since focusing to remain in a position and hold it requires concentration, during which the mind controls the performance of the body, resulting in physical fitness and emotional stability. Furthermore, there are chemicals released in our blood stream responsible for the way we feel after yoga practice. The journal of psychiatry and neuroscience describes yoga as a natural way to increase serotonin, which reduces depression. Endorphins, gamma-aminobutyric acid, and dopamine, which are released by the brain, all contribute to lowering stress and restoring peace.

When I do yoga, I pay attention to my body, and I do as much as it allows me to do. I have improved over the years, but I have not reached an advanced level, which is perfectly fine.

    h. Meditation – Similar to yoga, meditation is a marvelous activity for the mind and the body. In simple meditation you can use solely the power of your breath while being in a sitting position.

I enjoy Buddha-style sitting with crossed legs for at least fifteen minutes. There are different lotus positions for crossing your legs, and it is best to choose the one that is most comfortable for you.

Meditation is a practice of eliminating the clutter in your head and stopping your mind from wandering in different directions. It calls for you to pay attention to your breath and focus your mind on something pleasing, like a beautiful scene from your travels or a picture you love. Some practices even include music to soothe your mind. In meditation you will be aware of your feelings, your body, and your thoughts while slowing down the processes of engagement as an outsider simply watching them. Mindfulness of your general physical and emotional state will surface, and it is an introspective awareness that will keep you in check if you are not focused on the proper image or object. This is the simplest of practice that I am sharing for dealing with the stress of everyday life. I usually meditate in the morning in a cross-legged position with coffee in my hand. My mind chooses a favorite scene, such as snorkeling amidst colorful beautiful fish or standing on top of a mountain. This is the time of the day when I love being in the present moment, focusing on my breath or watching my thoughts. This simple practice helps me to be serene and peaceful for the rest of the day.

Antonina Duridanova

Singing, dancing, and playing a musical instrument are activities that produce indescribable feelings of joy, inner satisfaction, excitement, and happiness. I was exposed to singing and dancing at an early age. When I was four or five, my aunt organized gatherings at our apartment in Sofia, at which she loved to sing. Her deep voice touched the heart with the words and the melodies of her songs. She had a friend who sang with her, which made the songs more melodious and beautiful. I used to sit with an open mouth, very much touched and impressed with my aunt's talent. Later, she married a Macedonian, who was a very cheerful guy, always with a smile and singing as soon as he walked in the door. I started to sing later while attending an English language preschool program. This was a group singing exercise where everybody followed the music of the accordion played by our music teacher. I used to run home and sing all the songs I learned to the family; some of the songs I still remember and hum, or whistle. They continue to have the same joyous effect on me, making me smile and taking me back to my childhood. Music was a mandatory subject in Bulgaria, with music theory and singing, and I was very excited to learn the notes of the songs that we sang. Later, I sang in the high school choir, which I looked forward to with great enthusiasm. And I loved memorizing and singing the Beatles songs to my friends, which they found to be awesome. Years later when I was fifty-nine, I joined a Bulgarian folk singing group in San Antonio and we had a performance at a library in front of friends and visitors. What made this event special was that my daughter Vanesa was also singing in the choir.

14

Music is an important part of my life. I dreamt of playing the piano all my life, and one of the first things I did when I retired was buy a piano and start taking piano lessons. I love to sing or hum when I play the piano. It is a sublime experience which disconnects me completely from the outside world. Playing the piano is an enormous physical and mental exercise as it requires exclusive concentration and coordination of fingers moving on the keyboard with recognition of notes and accompanied by movements of the foot on the pedal. The music I like varies from classical to folk, rock, dance, and popular. I also like to attend music concerts of all music genres. When I listen to instrumental music, I transport myself in the world of the composer. I am particularly fond of Peruvian pan flute tunes. And I have always preferred music that makes me want to dance.

It is comprehensive why feelings connected with singing and playing musical instruments affect us. The same "happy" chemicals mentioned previously in connection with exercise and meditation—endorphins serotonin and dopamine are released in the blood when we listen to music. Singing is sometimes referred to as an aerobic activity because of the oxygen released in our system, which increases blood circulation. When we sing, our lungs expand, and the muscles around the ribcage are activated, resulting in increased lung capacity. Besides serving as a stress relief exercise, singing improves memory, because we need to remember the words of the song while singing in tune to the music. Songs are used to stimulate emotions and carry messages, letting people express their feelings and act in certain ways. They can motivate, mobilize to be more productive, as well as help with falling asleep. Playing the piano has valuable benefits for my body and mind as it requires intense concentration in performing associated with movements of the hands, fingers, wrists, eyes, head, and feet. And every time I learn to play a new piece of music, I feel enormous pleasure and joy.

Dancing is very much connected to singing as it is stimulated by the songs or melodies we hear, and the ones we like make us start tapping our feet, dancing in our seat, and finally, jumping and moving to the music.

My dancing experience started at an early age at the gatherings that my aunt organized, the same ones at which I learned to love singing. In those days in the mid-1950s, the adults in Bulgaria danced tangoes and waltzes. I was fascinated by the gracious movements of both dances and tried to imitate them to the rhythm of the music. When my aunt saw that, she took me by the hand and showed me the steps taking me into the fascinating world of dancing.

Much later as a teenager in an Eastern European communist country where western music and dancing were forbidden, I started to get together with classmates at private parties to dance the Twist—somehow the dance has penetrated the Iron Curtain and was extremely popular among the young people. I remember losing myself in swaying and twisting my body, and occasionally adding certain movements for fun. Once during summer vacation with mom at the Black Sea in the city of Balchik, I noticed on the way to the beach a flyer announcing a dance contest at one of the restaurants. That evening I snuck out and went to the designated place from the flyer. Standing in the middle of the dance floor I was approached by a boy (I was sixteen at the time) and asked to be his dance partner. And we danced away like we were one, swept by the music and enjoying every move. At the end of the contest, we both sat down at a table in the front, out of breath and all in sweat, anxiously waiting for the contest results.

We won first place, and everybody was clapping as we received a flower bouquet and a bottle of champagne. The boy smiled and said: "Take them both as you deserve the prize. I could not have done it alone." It was getting late, and I was becoming nervous returning to the house where we stayed. It was a vacation arrangement from my mother's work, and we were sharing a room with two other women. Approaching the house, I saw Mom walking down the street towards me, and I could tell even from a distance that she was upset. "Mom, Mom!" I started to shout. "I won a dance contest. I was at the restaurant that had the event, and this is what they gave me." I could tell that Mom was hesitating whether to scold me or congratulate me. "Don't disappear like that anymore," was all she said.

She took the bottle of champagne to share with the other women who congratulated me for winning a dance contest.

When I was in high school, I regularly met with my classmates on weekends to listen to the music of the sixties and dance. And when I was a college student in Belgrade, Yugoslavia, I did not miss a night of dancing at the students' club.

As adult I joined a gym, and I included in my routine Zumba and aerobics classes. I even talked my husband into enrolling in a dance class, to learn how to dance tango before we traveled to Argentina. Currently I am the oldest member of a Bulgarian folk dancing group in San Antonio. Bulgarian folk dancing features uneven beats and provides the best aerobic workout and mental exercise, because one needs to remember the constantly changing dynamic dance steps. It has been documented that the individual beats can be at a speed of 520 per minute. Performing on stage for different events in the city has been a big thrill because of the excitement, the public cheering, and the bonding with the young women in the group.

For me, dancing is the ultimate expression of happiness, where I get lost to the sounds and rhythm of music, forgetting all cares in the world. I do not need researchers to tell me that dancing is good for me emotionally and physically as I feel so good and toned up after dancing. And these effects are due to heavy doses of dopamine released in our system causing us to experience extreme pleasure; serotonin lowers the levels of depression and endorphins like dopamine contribute to the experience of pleasure. Added is the release of oxytocin because of the closeness to another person.

The following is a list of activities which I follow during the week.
- Walking – everyday morning or evening, moderate pace, thirty minutes to an hour
- Hiking – once a week one or two hours at moderate pace, weekday, or weekend

- Yoga – three to four times a week, thirty minutes to an hour, fifteen minutes of yoga every day
- Biking – every second day for forty to fifty minutes
- Dancing – Bulgarian folk dancing – once a week for an hour
- Swimming – every second day, weather permitting, ten to twelve laps

Every morning I select a couple of exercises and ensure that I do them at preferable times, coordinating with my mental activities—cooking, playing the piano, writing, painting, and language lessons.

When on vacation I adjust my routine to include more walking, hiking, snorkeling, and kayaking if by the sea. For example, at Cinque Terre, we hiked three days in a roll from one village to another, admiring spectacular views of the sea and the countryside as well as the scenic villages as we approached them.

CHAPTER 2
Nutrition

My diet is healthy and enjoyable, consisting of tasty dishes that provide the necessary nutrition to sustain a happy and pleasant life. Included in the appendix are some of my favorite recipes. I largely follow the diet that I enjoyed as a child, consisting of meals with fresh vegetables and fruits, fish, chicken, and occasional red meat. I eat healthily because of the way my grandmother raised me. She cooked with vegetables from the garden in her village, which she canned for the winter. Bulgarian food is like Mediterranean, somewhat Greek, and Turkish, with emphasis on fruits and vegetables. I passed my grandmother's and mother's recipes on to my children, and my daughters are constantly looking for more recipes from the Balkan Peninsula. My son's cooking, besides based on fresh produce, is gourmet style. My daughter in Kentucky has an acre of a garden, as she remembered how Bulgarians grow vegetables in the villages to manage on tight budgets. And my oldest daughter in San Antonio sends me daily recipes of healthy food, which we sometimes cook together.

I do not believe in diet programs where people torture themselves to follow a program in counting carbs and calories, and ordering special foods which are cooked with nobody knows what ingredients, additives, and preservatives. My solution to a healthy diet is to prepare my own meals and know their ingredients. Occasionally, I go out to eat, and when I travel, I eat mostly fruits and vegetables.

Examples of criteria which people consider when choosing food:

1. Appearance or the way the food looks like – When we were at the street night market in Kyoto, I admired the stalls where the food was displayed and arranged so esthetically, so colorfully,

that I had to try some of the snacks, which were not only good looking but also delicious. I will never forget that experience. Even now I can find the place if I am in Kyoto. There was counter after counter that resembled more like art displayed in a gallery than food in a marketplace.

2. Smell – When I am biking in the neighborhood on weekends, I can always smell the barbecue, and even if I am not hungry, I feel like going home and cooking.

And when I walk down a street with restaurants, the smell makes me want to stop and have a bite. When traveling in Europe in the summer, my best dining experiences were at places where the smell of food made me salivate.

3. Habit and experience – If somebody mentions to me *moussaka, banitsa, tarator,* "*kebapche,* I immediately imagine how the food looks like and how it tastes. I will order any of those Bulgarian dishes without even seeing them. (The appendix has recipes for these meals).

Nourishment is habit-forming. When babies are born and growing, they are introduced to different foods by their parents. I remember my daughter-in-law saying about my granddaughter: "I can't believe it; she loves everything I give her. Today she had avocado." Children's taste for food changes as they grow up. My grandchildren twins in Kentucky who are twelve turned up their noses to avocado, saying that it was mushy. When I lived in Ann Arbor, Michigan, we went to a Mexican restaurant, and my first experience was not that good. But now, living in San Antonio, Texas, and after numerous visits to Mexico, I find Mexican food delicious. I have found out that it is best to give food a chance and experiment with it. In the last twenty years I have learned to like not only European food but also African, Latin American, and Asian. My selections are still based on preferences I have had since childhood. I choose food with more vegetables, soups, and salads, and I also added to my diet healthier spices like turmeric and ginger.

Magic for Longevity: How I Stay Fit, Healthy and Happy

Proper nourishment is recognized as a big factor for fitness and longevity, and ideally, it starts at an early age, when our bodies are craving vitamins and food to grow. We need the right food to help us stay energetic, vigorous, and in good condition. I was fortunate to have a healthy food regime from an early age. I grew up in Bulgaria, where the food we ate changed with the seasons. The Balkan Peninsula diet is much talked about today because of its use of vegetables, olive oil, garlic, and onions as essential ingredients. In the summer we ate meals prepared with fresh vegetables from my grandmother's village. And in each season, we had specific fruits. There were strawberries and cherries in the spring; peaches, apricots, watermelons in the summer; and grapes in the fall. Eating fresh seasonal fruits and vegetables is not only tasty but also nutritious because they contain vitamins and minerals developed in the natural environment. Besides, our bodies need certain foods when transitioning into seasons. We crave berries, watermelons, peaches, salads in the summer, all of which help to keep us hydrated. I will never forget the tasty, delicious oranges from the farms in central Florida. They were sweeter, juicier, and tastier than the oranges we buy anywhere in the stores. In September and October my grandma canned red peppers and other vegetables; filled a barrel with cabbage, turning into sauerkraut for the winter. Recent studies talk about the nutritional value of sauerkraut, with its lactobacilli bacteria for preventing colds in the winter. Our diet also included daily Bulgarian yogurt, which is known for its bacteria bulgaricus, isolated in Bulgaria. Yogurt is known to help the immune and digestive systems. White bread was expensive, so we ate only rye bread, which was another plus, since studies show that white bread is not so healthy. Seasonal eating is a topic discussed nowadays, but in the past was a way of living—the food that we prepared was the food that was available for the season.

My current diet has changed somewhat since fresh vegetables and fruits are now available year-round. But I still cook sauerkraut and beans in the winter and use frozen berries and dried fruits for dessert. I am not a nutritionist, and I do not follow anybody's diet, but the meals I prepare

are recipes I learned from my childhood with abundant use of vegetables and less meat. I am not vegetarian, and our diet includes veal, lamb, chicken, and occasional beef, but the meat I use is for flavor and not the main course. My meal will consist of colorful vegetables, which provide different vitamins and minerals.

My daily food regime starts with a cup of coffee and a small bowl of yogurt with any available fruit—berries, kiwi, banana, mango, or papaya. Lunch consists of salads—lettuce (all kinds), cucumbers, tomatoes, avocado, corn, mango, papaya; or meals prepared with vegetables—green beans, carrots, mushrooms, eggplants, cabbage, peppers, tomatoes, broccoli, sprouts, asparagus, and corn; and fish and meat are optional. Dinner is light—toast with smoked salmon, grilled vegetables, or a slice of pizza with vegetables (spinach, artichoke, peppers, onion, mushrooms, Parmesan), a slice of *banitsa*, crepe, fruits, cheeses, or oatmeal.

Here are some of the herbs I use:

1. Spices – turmeric, cumin, black and white pepper, allspice, paprika, coriander, oregano, summer savory, and sea salt, which I prefer because of its enhanced taste and its healthy attributes of sodium chloride, known to regulate the fluid balance and blood pressure, as well as minerals such as potassium, iron, and calcium.

2. Herbs – parsley, dill, cilantro, rosemary, thyme, basil, bay leaf, lemongrass, mint, and ginger.

CHAPTER 3
Learned Behavior And Habits

This book will show how we need to constantly adjust our habits or learned behavior to continue living a healthy and happy life. As we age, our metabolism slows down, and we need to adjust our diet as well as our exercise routine. I stopped eating breakfast when I was not hungry in the morning. When I worked outside of the house, we had a big dinner in the evening, which now I have replaced with healthy snacks—yoghurt and fruit.

Exercising was not on my mind when I was in my twenties. I was active without keeping track of my daily activities. I noticed that in my mid-thirties I needed to start a workout program and watch my diet. I joined a gym, which I visited daily; I swam, did a cycle of weightlifting, and participated in aerobic group exercises. I trimmed the portion of my meals, and after a month, when I achieved my desired results, I reduced my visits to the gym to twice or three times weekly and increased to a certain degree the amount of my food intake, keeping an eye on my weight every day.

Changing my habits and routine was necessary because gaining weight of twenty pounds after giving birth to Anabelle at the age of thirty-four made me feel sluggish and slowed me down. Joining a gym which I regularly visited and changing my diet helped me lose weight and feel well and energetic. Ever since then I adopted a new style of living where I include physical exercises in my daily activities.

Adjusting to a program of daily exercises was not difficult for me as I have habits from my childhood to stay active and to eat healthy. Nonetheless, occasionally I fall into temptation of having a hamburger, French fries, or other fast food. Now I seldom have a taco for breakfast, or burger for lunch. What I found out is that if you eat healthy meals of quality and tasty food, this urge for a burger or hot dog eventually fades away. What is important is to realize that we need to change our diet at a certain age to have a healthy mind and body.

CHAPTER 4
Weight Control

Weight control is nowadays a very popular topic. Being on the go, we are all tempted to grab a burger, fries, or any other fast food. I know there are people making a conscientious effort to eat healthily by ordering salads and avoiding all their favorite foods, like popcorn at work. In my experience eating fast food once in two months or so does not impact my health or how I feel, provided I eat sensibly by including most of the time in my diet as many vegetables and fruits as possible. I am not following any specific diet, counting calories and carbs. What I do is regulate the portion of food in my dish and the kind of drink that accompanies it. When I was in my twenties, I had no trouble going back to my original shape and weight almost immediately and without any effort after I gave birth to my son and daughter. But when I had my second daughter at age thirty-four, the pounds and fat around my belly did not go away on their own. I felt sluggish and did not like how I looked. That was when I joined a gym, attended it every evening after work, and adopted a diet of no breakfast, green salad, radishes, and boiled egg for lunch, and a dinner one quarter of the regular size of a meal that was served to everybody else at home.

Breakfast is said to be the most important meal of the day, and that may be true for construction workers or farmers, but I am never hungry in the morning. Cutting out breakfast and changing other meal preferences combined with exercising helped me lose twenty pounds, and I have not gained it back since that time. My weight might go up and down a few pounds, but that is easily manageable.

I am not a fan of soft drinks, which I rarely have, and I drink a lot of water. I like an occasional glass of wine with my main meal, and every now and then a shot of whiskey, rakiya, or tequila. Another important thing about the way we treat food and drinks is that sometimes it is based on emotions. Some people lose their appetite when they are having issues or problems, others start eating uncontrollably or turn to alcohol or drugs. That is as destructive as it can be because problems do not go away; in fact, they become worse. Being intoxicated, obese, or anorexic could lead to severe health issues. Life problems are resolved with a clear mind and by engaging in some healthy activities such as exercise, reading a book, or travel.

I still remember my great-grandfather in my grandmother's village who was over hundred years old. He always started the day with a shot of rakiya. And, of course, all the meals for the day were prepared from food grown on the farm. He would sit outside under the shade of a tree and watch everybody doing their chores. I am sure his lifestyle in the country contributed to his living to be one hundred years old. The family moved later to the city but kept its ties to the countryside as we continued to visit and join in the daily farm activities. The lesson I learned from those days is that it is very important not to lose touch with nature and to enjoy all the benefits that it has to offer.

These are basic steps that I take for weight management:

1. I weigh myself first thing in the morning and before bedtime. In this way I know if I need to adjust my meals on the next day.
2. I never eat when I am not hungry.
3. In the morning, I eat or make a slush drink of yogurt and fruits.
4. For lunch I eat salads and soups, or dishes with predominantly vegetables.
5. I have a light dinner and avoid eating past 6:00 p.m.

CHAPTER 5
Lifestyle And Our Frame Of Mind

We choose the way we live by studying and accumulating knowledge which helps us realize our dreams. I immigrated from communist Bulgaria to be free and to have an opportunity to choose what to study and what kind of life to live. I have three college degrees, which led to a very glamourous career which made me feel self-fulfilled and happy. It also helped me raise three children and take care of my mother. A successful career guarantees financial security, which provides us with a comfortable living, free of stress and worries about our livelihood. It gives us freedom to choose where to live, travel, and how to spend our free time. I worked hard, and my reward was that when I retired, I was able to pick up activities that I like. I started to play the piano, paint, and travel. I write books and have book events at which I meet wonderful people.

Financial stability also affects our emotional state, as it puts us in control of our destiny.

An important point to keep in mind is that the way we are conditioned to think and perceive that the outside world is what impacts our lives. Positive thinking is the key to success, as it allows us to keep a clear head and stay focused when pursuing a goal. Learning to deal with issues in an organized and calm manner is important for sustaining a healthy body and mind. Self-control in evaluating situations and taking correct decisions is essential for overcoming tough times and moving forward to a brighter life. In my personal experience I had to deal with unpleasant situations, which I resolved by confronting the issues and following a plan for their resolution. My view on life is that you need to feel free to create, to express your thoughts, to continuously learn and pursue new goals. The ultimate satisfaction you obtain from life is based on your efforts, resilience, perseverance, and determination to reach your goal. You are the only boss of your destiny, and the choices you make determine the course of your life.

CHAPTER 6
Mind-Exercising Activities

The physical exercises which I described in an earlier chapter also influence our minds. However, it is worth discussing solely mind-engaging exercises, which in turn affect our physical state.

STUDYING LANGUAGES

The benefits of learning languages are significant. Studying a language improves concentration and memory because it requires you to remember and use foreign words and compose a sentence in a different order than we are used to. Since every language has its own patterns and structures, studying a language improves problem solving, decision making, multitasking, and listening skills. It also contributes to creative thinking and better concentration. But what is most valuable is that communication with people of different cultures enhances our understanding of the world and opens windows to unimaginable possibilities of learning and appreciating diverse customs and ways of living.

The most important thing is that speaking a language allows us to connect with people from all over the world and when traveling to be able to get oriented and easier in an unknown environment. Knowing a language is also useful when working in a foreign country. One of my degrees is in French and Russian languages and literature, and while on a book tour in Bulgaria with my book *New Beginnings: From Behind the Iron Curtain to America*, a journalist asked me why I studied Russian, since I escaped from the Soviet-dominated regime in Bulgaria. My answer was that during an assignment to Moscow as a tax advisor after the fall of communism, I could communicate directly with officials from the Russian Ministry and write my reports in Russian, which facilitated my work. Knowing French, I could speak with representatives of the European Union from France, which was appreciated, and it also helped me to establish a better working relationship with my counterparts from Europe. My master's degree is in International Business and Spanish Language. Spanish is useful when communicating with Spanish-speaking people in my current city as well as when traveling to Spain and Latin America. Currently, I take lessons in Chinese, a fascinating language with amazing culture. For example, adults never make negative comments or insult another person in public, something the Western world should work on, as destructive behavior has adverse effects on us, not to mention the display of ridiculous and embarrassing behavior.

Chinese language is challenging as same words have completely different meanings based on their intonation. Word structure has nothing to do with any of the Roman, Germanic, or Slavic group languages that I am familiar with. Writing with characters is like painting five hundred basic characters, which I decided to keep at a minimum and rely on Pinyin—roman letters with accents for word pronunciation. People asked me why I study Chinese, and whether I intend to travel there. We traveled to Shanghai and Beijing prior to the COVID pandemic, and I was very much impressed with life in these cities, which I describe later in this book. But I do not have any practical reason for studying Chinese. What I receive from studying Chinese are the above-mentioned benefits. Besides, most of us start to lose our ability to remember as we age, and I have noticed that by studying Chinese and keeping up with the other languages that I know keeps my mind as sharp as it was twenty years ago. The added benefit is that it makes me happy to communicate with my Chinese teacher and friends from all other nationalities.

PLAYING A MUSICAL INSTRUMENT

I already talked about the physical benefits of playing the piano, but the most important part of it is the mental ability to concentrate on producing a tune, a song, a melody which is recognizable and provides pleasure when listening to it. I prefer taking lessons in person to those on the internet as I need interaction with my teacher to receive immediate reinforcement and feedback. I am patient with new songs as I study a couple of lines at a time, using first the right hand before adding the left and the pedal. What I discovered is that I need to practice the old songs every day for an hour or so, but I also want to be challenged learning new compositions. Playing the piano has become a part of my daily life and routine, as I cannot imagine the world without music.

READING AND WRITING

Reading is a mental exercise that takes you to other worlds and amazing places, which are real and imagined, and lets you peek into the lives of people. Reading helps us escape from reality and visit enchanting lands and appealing landscapes, as well as become a part of the characters' lives. Sometimes we can identify with them or just be entertained by the twists and turns in a story of mystery, romance, or real-life experiences. I started to read when I was seven, as this was the age for starting school in Bulgaria, but I fell in love with books when I was two or three, listening to my aunt reading the Hans Christian Anderson or the Thousand-and-One-Night stories at bedtime. And when I learned to read, I read every book for kids of my age in the local library.

Reading can slow down the hustle and buzzle of your life, introduce peace and tranquility, increase your knowledge in history, geography, psychology, science and entertain you with literary fiction of mystery, romance, horror, poetry, drama, art, photography, travel, and humor. Most importantly it helps you develop your imagination.

Writing is another activity which enhances the brain's functions as a great mental exercise, which invokes creativity and the ability to sort out and remember facts. Writing your memoir and biography helps you recollect moments of your past. Fellow writers of fiction stories share with me that writing stimulates their imagination and creativity. I also discovered that writing enables me to be organized and focused on resolving issues. In searching for new words, synonyms, etc., my vocabulary has increased, which in turn has improved my communication and logical skills. It also helps me keep a clear mind and stay alert.

I became serious about writing my memoir during the COVID pandemic, and in a couple of months I was ready to have it edited by a friend, who was an English major. Shortly thereafter I researched on Google and came across a publisher, Fulton Books, which I immediately contacted. A couple of days later I received a call which made me very happy. They accepted to publish my book; memoir titled *New Beginnings: From behind the Iron Curtain to America*. My life has changed drastically since the publishing of my book, which was also translated and published in Bulgarian, my native language. What touches me the most is that I reach the hearts of my readers with my message that people should be courageous to overcome all difficulties and follow their dreams. It also made my American readers reflect on their lives and appreciate the freedom and opportunities they have in America. Participating in numerous book events at bookstores, libraries, and festivals in America and in Bulgaria, book bazars at the Bulgarian Cultural Centers in Chicago, giving workshops at universities and schools provides me utmost pleasure. Interviews that I gave to programs of the Bulgarian National Radio and television and journalists of magazines and newspapers are very memorable and self-gratifying experiences as I continue educating and inspiring people of all ages.

CHAPTER 7
Friendship

Life is more enjoyable with friends. This is a proven fact in my life. My friends and I share our lives, experiences, thoughts, and ideas. We celebrate good times and achievements in person and virtually, and we support each other in tough times. I lost touch with a lot of my friends because of relocating. Even with social media I cannot find classmates from the English Language High School in Sofia, the Economics Faculty in Belgrade, or even people I met on my journey immigrating from Bulgaria and arriving in Ann Arbor, Michigan.

I currently live in San Antonio Texas, and I am happy to have in the city friends and coworkers from my work. I also met Bulgarians who live in Texas and joined their folk-dance group. Celebrating Bulgarian and American holidays and attending gatherings in the company of people from my homeland is essential to keep me in touch with my origin and my roots.

I also met my husband's friends. His fellow doctor, who happened to be a former neighbor from my hometown; a painter and her husband; a Brazilian lady; and other of his colleagues and acquaintances added to the circle of our friends.

I also have had the incredible opportunity of meeting wonderful people in the States and in Europe since the publication of my book. I joined university and women organizations, international book clubs and societies where I met exceptional individuals with similar interests and ideas. My ultimate joy is when I participate at book bazars and cultural activities at the Bulgarian Cultural Centers in Chicago, and other American cities, meeting with principals of Bulgarian schools in America and sharing topics of history with Bulgarian children. I expanded my presentations by offering workshops at American universities and schools, which I tremendously enjoy as communicating with young people and inspiring them to reach their goals is very gratifying for me. My life is rich and meaningful, surrounded by so many old and new friends who offer their love and support with comments about my book. Some of my readers remember their childhood with the games we played, others recall the reality of growing up during the communist regime with restrictions on travel, and whatsoever news from the West. I felt extremely happy when I heard that my book also helped folks overcome difficult personal and professional times. Then there are readers who feel that I had a mission to complete returning to Bulgaria after the fall of communism as a US tax advisor to aid with the creation of a new Tax Administration, capable of functioning in a free market economy. My readers in America share how blessed they feel that they were born in America where they are free and have tremendous opportunities to grow and develop. All my readers who crossed my path became my friends with whom I continue to stay in touch.

My ultimate reward was traveling to Bulgaria for the presentation of my book in Bulgarian language. Reconnecting with people whom I worked with as a tax advisor, especially the official from the Bulgarian Government who selected me to provide a tax reform assistance, was an extremely emotional experience. Spending time with relatives and friends was also very touching. I am looking forward to my next trip to Europe when I will reunite with people who are an important part of my life.

I want to mention that I appreciate social media as this is how I stay in touch with everybody and plan my visits and travel. In conclusion I cannot stress enough how important friendship is to me. All my friends in America and other places in the world play an important role in my life. They all provide me with a sense of belonging and a feeling of being loved. I gain from them comfort and strength as we share and exchange ideas, thoughts, interests, and give each other support. I would like to add that I recently read in Neuroscience and Biobehavioral Reviews of May 2020 that loneliness and living in seclusion can cause inflammation, leading to serious heart conditions, stroke, etc., as well as depression, which explains our need for friendship.

Social media is great to help us stay in touch but face-to-face meetings with friends are irreplaceable as a condition to live a healthy and happy life.

SUMMARY: PART ONE

I hope you enjoyed the first part of my book, and that I provided answers to your questions about what I do to preserve my vitality, appearance, and sharp mind. Most significant is to know how to alternate physical and mind exercises, and how to select your meals in order to have a grip on your strength and energy during the day. The information that I share is described in a very comprehensive way and it addresses various aspects of my activities and mindset to live a happy and healthy life. What I consider important is to take pleasure in everything you do from hiking in the park to walking on the beach or having a delicious meal with family and friends.

Here is a capture of my practices that help me to be healthy and happy:

1. Nutrition – I skip breakfast because I do not perform physical work; a drink of various fruits combined with coconut milk or yogurt is sufficient. I also drink a cup of coffee or tea to pick me up and to start my day on a happy note. For lunch I eat salads and soup, if I expect to work in the afternoon. I discovered that green salads and fish give me mental and physical energy, and I perform better when I include them in my midday meal. I do not eat dinner past 6:00 p.m. If there is a gathering in the evening, I limit what I consume to small appetizers. My main meal includes primarily vegetables—asparagus, broccoli, green beans, peppers, peas, corn, okra, eggplant, celery, carrots, onions, garlic, etc. I grew up in Bulgaria, and Bulgarian recipes have ingredients that are mostly vegetables with Mediterranean spices and a smitch of meat. Onions and garlic are the basis for my dishes. My soups can be creamy vegetables or soups, with seafood, chicken, pozole, beans, lentils, etc. I drink plenty of water, juices, lactose free, or almond milk. I rarely

drink carbonated drinks. I never buy them, but I do not exclude them completely as I remember once I had a sun stroke, and nothing helped my headache except a can of regular Coca-Cola. I use vitamins and supplements, such as Vitamin C, D, and Zinc, but not daily. I increase their intake in times of epidemics and flu seasons. I plan my meals and I store leftovers, some of which I incorporate in new recipes. For example, leftovers of vegetables and meat I bake in small clay pots with springled feta cheese and an egg on top for ten to fifteen minutes. I also use recipes from the internet to create an exciting and appealing menu. We traveled the world, and I introduce Thai, Chinese, Moroccan, and other countries meals in our diet. I eat out occasionally or when there is a special occasion for celebrating an event or meeting a friend.

2. Physical activity – My physical activity also varies and depends on the weather or the location, but I try to include a couple of activities during the day, and one of them is yoga. When I am at home, I alternate my activities of bike riding, walking, hiking, etc. as I have discovered that the use of different muscle groups during the week contributes to my overall feeling of being energetic and lively. I do not adhere to rigid schedules, which adds to the pleasure of my exercising. What matters is that at the end of the day I know that I have completed a healthy activity program as I feel strong and happy. Remember from my detailed discussions the chemicals that are released in the blood stream when exercising!

3. Mental exercises – I knew exactly what I was going to do when I retired. I bought a piano, then canvasses and paint supplies. Music makes me forget the outside world. Emotions overcome me and melodies touch my soul. For example, opera music reminds me of my mother, and I see myself sitting with her in the opera house in Sofia. Since I started to play piano, I feel happy when I learn how to play a new piece of music.

Playing the piano also requires a lot of concentration—notes recognition, finding the notes on the keyboard, using the correct fingers to play them, and counting. The combination of numerous mental and physical activities contributes to keeping a sharp mind and body.

My second passion, which is painting, transports me to another world. When I paint, I am immersed in creating a scene of a landscape or images by selecting the proper colors and shades that reproduce what I envision from my imagination or my travels. I find myself in a world of creativity, constantly problem solving to succeed in creating a final product, which delivers messages and meaning designed for my viewers.

Writing always fascinated me as a vehicle of communicating my thoughts, my beliefs, my values, and principles that I learned in early childhood from my grandmother in the Bulgarian countryside. I published my first book when I was seventy-one and received the utmost pleasure when I succeeded in delivering to my readers messages about the value of freedom and appreciation of life in America and the free world. This experience of connecting with my readers all over the world is priceless and the best reward I could receive in contributing to peace and understanding the true meaning of life.

Friends and relatives are essential for our existence. The smile on the faces of my children and grandchildren, their achievements, are the primary source of pleasure and enjoyment in my life.

I travel extensively, which increased after the debut of my book with book tours nationally and abroad, during which I met wonderful and amazing people. They all became my friends, embracing the values of freedom and an accomplished life for realization of dreams. My readers are a part of my life, my happiness and joy. I cherish every single contact with them, and I am delighted to see how my book serves as an inspiration for overcoming difficult situations as well as a guide to successfully reach one's goals.

My relationship with friends and family is reciprocal for support and advice, and this closeness is the driving source in my life. My family and friends from both sides of the ocean are a very important part of my life, as everything I do is meaningful because of them.

1. Short and long-term goals

I grew up in a family of intellectuals and developed my love for books at an early age. When I was young, I loved to study and learn in depth all the material in the school subjects. I graduated from an English Language High School in Bulgaria and continued my education after I immigrated to America. I am grateful for all the opportunities that my new home provided me. I loved studying foreign languages and economics, and I have degrees in Russian and French languages and literature, Business Administration, with a major in Accounting and a master's in International Business and Spanish. The education that I received led to my successful career with United States Treasury and an assignment, which was a realization of my dreams. I was appointed a United States tax advisor to Bulgaria after the fall of communism.

2. Here is an example of my current short- and long-term goals:
   a. Short-Term – Publish and release my second book in English and Bulgarian languages with presentations and interviews. Continue to have book events at schools and universities based on topics of my debut book.
   b. Long-term – Film making of my first book.
   Improve my piano playing and my Chinese language speaking skills. Improve my painting skills.
   Continue to travel and collect memories of places in Europe, Asia, Africa, and South America. I have already visited countries all over the world, and now I prefer to explore life in small villages.

My last comment is that a prerequisite for a happy life is to have the freedom to be engaged in activities that are important to you.

CHAPTER 8
Dealing With Transition

We undergo transitions in our lives at different times—when we graduate and start our first dream job or change careers, when we relocate, get married and have children, retire, and so on.

My major recent transition in life was retirement. I am sharing this experience because a lot of people feel lost on the day they stop working.

The life I knew for a long time stopped existing on the day I retired. The phones stopped ringing, there were no emails, and nobody called to share issues or ask for advice or help.

In retrospect, maybe I should have traveled somewhere to distract myself, but I stayed home. On the first day of my retirement, I woke up at the same time as usual and stretched in bed. My body started to become alive with every movement I made to meet the day. However, I felt rare, as if something was very wrong and out of place. Nobody was calling to inform me of their case issues or family problems. It was quiet, exceptionally quiet, which struck me at once. I quickly jumped out of bed, took a very hot shower, brushed my body vigorously with a rose-smelling sponge in the hope that my mood would improve, which always worked before, but not this time. I had an urge to be outside, so in no time I was in my car on the way to a nearby mall. It was a very pleasant, sunny day in San Antonio, Texas, on December 1st, 2014. I could hear birds singing outside my open driver's side window, but something was missing. Arriving early at the mall, I parked in the empty parking lot and slowly strolled towards the open-air shopping area. The tropical vegetation bathing in the sun was a pleasant sight. The stores were closed, and very few people were out for a quick walk or run. I was not in a hurry. Walking slowly from one part of the outside mall to the other, I started to feel somewhat better. I didn't notice how time passed, and storekeepers started to pull up the shutters of the store windows and open the doors. I always liked the awakening of the city, the fresh air at dawn, and the first sounds of vehicles and people talking. The faces of the friendly ladies from the Sisley counter at Neiman Marcus came to mind. Cheerful and smiling, they always made me happy. I slowly entered the store, spotted the women, and waved at them. They noticed me and waved back with a smile. I felt good, maybe because of my past visits with them. I increased my pace and soon I was in one of their chairs, getting complimentary makeup. My cosmetologist noticed a difference in me but did not mention a word. I never liked it when asked questions about my feelings or disposition, and I appreciate the discretion of people not bothering me with awkward for me questions. My friends at the beauty counter kept quiet, and I was glad that they respected my privacy. The funny thing is that one of the synonyms for privacy in the word thesaurus is retirement.

After a while I told them that it was my first day of retirement and that I had come to the mall on impulse. I told them how I loved seeing their happy faces and they responded that they enjoyed my visits and the photos and information that I shared about my travels. I went on to explain how it felt strange to wake up and realize that all daily tasks had disappeared, that there were no more deadlines, issues to resolve, and meetings to attend. Then I thanked them for their kindness, explaining that visiting them this morning made me feel good.

The next day I woke up, afraid that the same feeling of emptiness and discomfort would return, but I was alright. I made myself coffee and drafted a list of things I always wanted to do but couldn't while working. I planned to purchase a piano and found a piano teacher. I researched painting and drawing classes offered by the school district. I remembered how colleagues and friends had asked me to write a book about my life. But most importantly, I was looking forward to spending time with my children and grandchildren.

COVID –
Coping With Difficult Situations

Outside factors can unexpectedly invade our lives and paralyze all our activities and life as we know it, which has a tremendous effect on our psychological and physical health. I was able to live through COVID global catastrophe without any mental scars or physical issues by adjusting my schedules and routines.

COVID turned the entire world upside down. Nothing was the way it used to be. When it spread out to become a pandemic in 2020, everybody held their breath. Countries were invaded with this invisible and, for some, deadly monster. People's lives were threatened and lost, with no known cure to save anyone. Shopping was restricted; schools and businesses, banks, and government agencies were closed. Activities were put on hold. Then, all social functions were restructured. School and college learning was done online; employees worked from home whenever possible; people had food delivered to their homes by Amazon and big food chains rather than going to the store. It was at that time that I became serious about finishing my first book, a memoir entitled *New Beginnings: From Behind the Iron Curtain to America*, which was published a year later. After I retired in 2014,

I thought about writing a book describing my life journey and the challenges and achievements in pursuit of my dreams and realizing my goals. I bought books on how to write fiction and non-fiction and wrote a couple of chapters about my childhood in communist Bulgaria. During COVID, I took this task seriously and wrote a couple of hours a day to finish the book in two months, hired a publisher (Fulton Books was the first I saw on Google, so I selected them), and started the editing process. Also, during COVID I continued with piano and Chinese language lessons online. I took an oil painting class with my teacher from the community center using Zoom. Since all gyms were closed, I used YouTube for yoga classes. I bought a new, more comfortable bike and used a route which I took every day. Evenings and weekends I walked in the neighborhood or the park with Mitt, who started to work online. Since I love cooking, I pulled from the internet a variety of recipes, spending every day a few hours in the kitchen. I had a very busy schedule, which I adjusted as necessary. The thing missing from my life was travel. When the COVID vaccine first came out in January 2021, I was very hesitant about getting it, but a few months later my son told me that I could not travel to see them in Michigan unless I was vaccinated, so I decided to overcome my initial fear and get vaccinated.

I hadn't seen my son, my daughter-in-law and the kids since the fall of 2019, and I missed them. The kids were growing so fast. Anderson was ten, and Lucy was a toddler. I was so excited that I scheduled to spend three weeks in the month of June 2021 with them in Holland, Michigan. I can't describe the joy I felt as my son picked me up from the airport in Grand Rapids, Michigan, and drove me to their new house in a beautiful golf community. As the front door opened, their black Labrador dog, Ziggy, flew out and, not knowing me, stood across the street, observing what was going on. I had a Winnie the Pooh stuffed animal for Lucy to make friends with her, and she smiled at me, seeing her favorite toy. I also dressed in a yellow dress, since I learned that she loves the yellow color. I smiled back at her and hugged my daughter-in-law, who had a big smile on her face, too. My son took me downstairs to show me my room, and with a twinkle in his eyes said: "This is your room, Ma; you can come here whenever you want and stay for as long as you like." My heart filled with so much joy hearing these words. I hugged him and told him how much this meant to me. My daughter-in-law and Lucy were also there, all smiley, with Ziggy and Jasper the cat, who were lined up to take part in the family happy occasion.

We had so much to catch up on, so in the morning I learned all about Lucy's activities and the things she loved. And of course, she had to demonstrate everything that her mom was explaining. "Lucy can recognize all letters of the alphabet in their order and associate them with the objects that they stand for." Lindsey started to talk, and Lucy, already knowing the alphabet, took the letter m and pointed at Mom, the letter n for me, Nana, the letters d and c for dog and cat.

My son joined us in the evening, and we all had barbecue on the terrace. Our mornings for the rest of my stay were fabulous as we took long walks and I ran with Lucy, Lindsey, and Ziggy on the golf course in the back of the house, throwing a ball for Ziggy to catch and watching him let Lucy get it first and fetch it to him.

Evenings were also special as my son cooked gourmet meals on the grill, with music playing in the background and everybody dancing. Anderson, my grandson, came in a week and joined us in all the fun. There was a visit to the zoo, for which Lindsey's mother accompanied us, and we all enjoyed watching the kids, especially Lucy, having a special interest in all animals, waving and talking to them. Lindsey's parents made me feel so welcomed, inviting us to dinner at their home on Lake Michigan and on a boat ride to the neighboring Grand Haven, which was an exclusively delightful experience. The sight along the way of homes tucked in between trees, bushes, and flowers and the wind caressing my face made me feel marvelous, but what was extra special was the excitement of the children. Lucy pointed at the water and the waves squealing with joy, and Anderson was extremely happy to be grandpa's co-captain. Watching the sunset from the sandy shores of Grand Haven, with the beautiful red lighthouse, was a perfect ending to a fabulous day surrounded by family.

On Lucy's second birthday, June 25th, my daughter-in-law dressed her in a beautiful lacy dress. Lucy knew that it was a special occasion and assumed an important look. There was a gathering with a few friends and Lindsey's parents, in a very intimate and warm atmosphere. It was a beautiful summer day, and we all sat at the dining table on the second-floor terrace for a birthday celebration with a special meal and cake. A friend of the family who is a professional photographer captured with her camera every moment of the day's festivities. The days were going by quickly, and I used every second to play and be with Lucy and Anderson. I went down slides, jumped on inflatables at an indoor place full of activities for children, swam in the neighboring pool next to Lucy, and watched her getting braver and braver in the water. I played football in the pool and ping pong at home with Anderson. We also had fun reading books, solving puzzles, and figuring out an educational robot I got for Lucy from the bookstore.

I loved my days, which began with Jasper the cat and Ziggy the pup waiting at the door in the morning for me to get up, then leaping into my room with joy. Next, there was morning coffee in the sunroom; running at the golf course with Lindsey, the kids, and Ziggy, who took his morning swim at a lake; picnic lunches in the playroom; specialty dinners; and evening walks, when Lucy and Anderson used their outdoor toys, bikes, and sport games. Lucy was already saying words and showing pride in her accomplishments every day. Still, it was Lucy's personality which made her unique. She knew how to express emotions, but at the same time behaved and followed Mom and Dad's rules.

Both of my grandchildren were very affectionate as we said good night before bedtime, but Lucy needed to have the entire family hug together and kiss. I developed a lifetime bond with the children as Lucy would take me by the hand and lead me to the playroom and Anderson would enjoy laughing at my comments while we played ping pong.

This was the time when my book *New Beginnings: From Behind the Iron Curtain to America* was published and available for purchase on Amazon and at bookstores all over the country. My daughter-in-law had a big surprise for me, as she introduced my book to her neighbors and friends prior to my arrival, and I met my first readers for book signing. My son also had a book for me to sign. This was a gesture that I truly valued and appreciated. And since I stayed for a while, I did get to hear comments about my book from my first readers of how lucky they felt, comparing their lives in America to mine growing up in a communist country and risking my life to reach freedom.

We did not say goodbye, as we booked a follow up trip to Vegas for my son's birthday in October.

After my trip to Michigan to visit with my son and his family, I visited with my daughter, Anabelle, and her children in Kentucky. I booked a flight to Lexington, and from there I drove to Lake Cumberland to meet them. I rented a house tucked in the woods with a wrapped-around screened porch and a pool across from it. There was a pool table on the second floor that the kids were especially happy to see. I promised them horseback riding, so we did that on the first day, followed by going to a waterpark with waves in pools and big slides. What I really enjoyed was Isabelle's giggling and the smile on her brothers' faces running from one slide to another. At Lake Cumberland I met the owner's wife, with whom I had coffee each morning. She loved hearing about my story described in the book. The entire complex was amazing, with houses hidden in the woods and several pools to accommodate all locations. The evenings were also very pleasant. I cooked and was happy to see that the kids liked my meals. Isabelle liked to draw, so she showed me how she used the internet to create her drawings. This trip was not long, but it was special, and I knew I would be returning for Anabelle's graduation in December, so nobody felt too sad saying goodbye.

I include this information about my life in semi-isolation due to COVID as a demonstration of how I adjusted to new restrictions and restructured my life to meet the demands of an extreme situation. During the first two years of COVID, there was a significant increase in depression because of isolation, physical sicknesses, and fear. Writing my book during

COVID opened a new world for me. I enjoyed being creative and meeting with authors, poets, journalists, and literary critics. I also met and was contacted by many people who read my book from both sides of the Atlantic Ocean, since my book was translated in Bulgarian language. Comments about the emotions that my book aroused in my readers made me very happy, feeling that I succeeded in delivering messages of survival and success. Balancing mental and physical activities during COVID enabled me to overcome negativity and avoid health problems.

I have shared details of my trip and visit with my son and his family because I believe that such contact with family is crucial for our health. Involvement in children's games, seeing how pleased they are with discovering new things, and how sincere they are in expressing emotions fills my heart with joy and pleasure.

I returned to Kentucky in December for Anabelle's graduation, which was a very important day in her life. For Anabelle, it was proof that she could achieve her goals with persistence, organization, and determination, even during the challenging time of COVID. Her community college conducted an intimate ceremony at a church with encouraging motivational speeches. What excited me was Jacob's and Isabelle's interest in following the ceremony on the stage and listening with curiosity, as I could tell by the expressions on their faces with wide open eyes. Anabelle's accomplishment gave my grandchildren the lesson I gave her, that learning is essential for success and happiness. It was an amazing feeling to be proud together with my grandchildren of my daughter's achievement.

I, as a mother, can feel my children's happiness or pain no matter how far they are. Their achievements are always a source of energy and strength for me.

In conclusion I would say that times spent with family and interactions with kids and grandkids have a tremendous impact on our mental state.

Being with family and offering and receiving support in times of pursuing goals is a very important part of our life. There is no value that can be placed on such a relationship.

CHAPTER 9
Spiritual Activities

ART – FOOD FOR THE SOUL

My love for art started at an early age when my mom took me to art galleries and taught me how to back up and look at paintings from a distance to better interpret what the painter was trying to convey. "Viewing a painting from a distance is the only way to enjoy it," she used to say, asking me to go close and far to compare the difference. We often visited a gallery in the city park, especially when there was a change of an exhibit. One of Mom's older students who became an artist used to visit her, and I started to draw with him, getting my first lessons in drawing and later in water coloring. It was then when I realized that drawing is a way to express your feelings. I drew white pigeons with the inscription "peace," just about the time when my parents were getting a divorce. I loved the time at my maternal grandmother's village, and I sketched the fields, wildflowers, butterflies, and farm animals.

We also had drawing and painting classes starting in elementary school. I remember in second grade the teacher placing an apple on her desk, saying that it had to be drawn by the end of the hour. "Antonina has talent, which needs to be developed," Mom's student used to say. But my parents, both intellectuals (Dad was a university professor and Mom a high school teacher), steered me away from becoming an artist. They were both determined that I needed a solid, serious career, and art, in their minds, was a hobby, not a career.

As time went by, I was so busy at the English language high school that I had no time for painting. Immigrating from communist Bulgaria at the age of nineteen, I received my higher education in America and eventually had a career with United States Treasury. I had a demanding position, and I was taking care of my children and my mother, which prevented me from being able to paint. It was after retirement that I started painting again. I was so happy when one of the gifts I received at my retirement party was acrylic paints, brushes, and a canvass. I was thrilled that I would learn how to paint with acrylics. Then it occurred to me that the hostess of our book club was a very talented painter. Her paintings were abstract, based on shapes and forms, sometimes delivering messages, and other times simply expressing the process of creating a composition based on a vision. I started to visit her and learned how to project an image from a photo on the much bigger canvass. She taught me how to mix paint and create different shades of one color. My first painting was a sunrise on a beach in Bali, a place that I loved because of its exotic and beautiful scenery and heartwarming people. My friend displayed my painting in her living room for everybody to see at our book club meeting, and people exclaimed saying how beautiful it was. "That's wonderful, Antonina," one woman said. "My first painting was of an apple, and you created a very attractive landscape."

The reaction of my friends gave me confidence to continue painting more landscapes that I loved from our trips. My second painting was from a hiking trip in Morea. I used a photo we took of the jungle overlooking the water. I was so excited that I was up in the middle of the night, mixing different shades of green to produce the desired green color for the foliage of the forest at the upper part of the hill, and the meadow at the bottom which extended to the sea.

The blue colors were easier to manage, and by morning I had completed the painting. I backed up to view it as Mom taught me to and was satisfied with the result. Both paintings are hung on the wall in the master bedroom on both sides of the bed frame.

Africa inspired me so much that I had to express my feelings on a canvass. We traveled twice to Africa, alongside the east and west coasts of the continent, and both times I was amazed by the tranquility and balance in nature. My first African painting portrayed images of animals that I saw on a safari near Cape Town, to which I added a crocodile from a place that we visited in Durban. My painting reproduced the harmony of life between elephants, lions, and crocodiles all in a natural habitat—the lions in bushes, under a tree; the elephants playing in a pond; and the crocodile in muddy water. I remember picking up acrylic paints to resemble colors of lions and crocodiles, which still needed mixing with similar other colors, and carefully selecting colors to reproduce the environment with hills in the back disappearing in the horizon.

On our trip to Botswana, I was extremely impressed with a herd of elephants coming to drink water in the Chobe River, a scene that I recreated when I returned home. For enhancement I added a monkey and other animals that I had seen during the day. Along the way by the river, I spotted the unusual sight of a crocodile and, nearby, a buffalo with a bird on him, who seemed to hesitate what to do with the crocodile. This painting I gave to my grandson Jorden as well as a painting of giraffes, which he chose, as a memory of his grandmother's treasured experience.

The safari trip in the desert in Dubai was an amazing experience, so I painted a man and a woman, which was supposed to be Mitt and myself, on a camel. Abu Dhabi's skyline dazzled me, which prompted me to paint its modern buildings.

Since I found out that acrylic paints dry fast, I wanted to learn how to use oil paints and signed up for the only oil painting class available at the time at the San Antonio Community Center, where I met my art teacher Maren. The class was fast paced, requiring the completion of two paintings in three hours. I sweated it a bit but succeeded in keeping up with the program. I discovered that oil paint does not dry fast and needs to be handled carefully. After experimenting with acrylic and oil paints, I must say that I prefer oil paints because the colors are more vivid and do not change after mixing. My painting from the canals of Amsterdam, a city that completely impressed me with its free spirit and beautiful scenery, hangs on the wall at my daughter's house, together with a scenery of a beautiful cave with gorgeous reflections from the sunlight and a waterfall in Kawai from a trip with my daughter Vanesa and her husband.

My son-in-law in San Antonio made me happy when he selected for his office paintings of a rooster and of a winter scene.

Another oil painting class, which I took online during COVID, allowed me to reproduce some of my favorite scenes from my travels, such as a street with old Bulgarian houses, the Venice canal, giraffes with the Kilimanjaro Mountain in the background, a mountain landscape with a river, and flowers and Taj Mahal—a challenging painting of this monument of love because of the precision and details in its architectural structure. However, my favorite oil painting is that of a street with old houses in Bulgaria, reminding me of the times I was with Mom in Koprivshtitsa. Every time I look at it, I can see Mom's smiling face taking my hand and the two of us walking down the cobblestone streets.

I also wanted to go back to watercolor painting, familiar to me from my childhood. I signed up for a class at the community center and was happy to see familiar faces from my earlier oil painting class. I found painting in a group very useful as we compared our paintings, expressed opinions, and offered one another advice on how to improve. Walking away from a painting and returning to it on the next day was a good idea, especially with watercolors as the paint of different colors can settle with time and give amazing results.

For the water coloring class, I chose to paint breathtaking landscapes from my recent travels. The paintings that I have on my family room wall are a scene from Machu Picchu, a remarkable place in the Andes Mountains, and a painting of the beautiful Bulgarian Rose Valley. I painted a Peruvian girl standing by a llama in the Machu Picchu mountains, and a girl in a Bulgarian folk dress outfit by a well with a balance beam (*kobilitsa*) to carry water to add authenticity to both paintings.

I continued to experiment drawing and painting and took another class of charcoal painting. Getting all the necessary supplies, I selected the compositions of places close to my heart. During a recent travel to Cabo San Lucas, I was impressed by a rock formation in the water known as the Arch, and I chose it for my drawing, connecting it with the experience of being on a sightseeing ship. I had a few other successful still-life drawings, and l was happy with my accomplishments.

Abstract painting always attracted me with its bold representations of figures in vivid colors. An Introduction to Abstract Painting class took me to another world of painting, during which I decided that I preferred abstract expressionism. My art teacher from the community center evaluated my paintings and concluded that I tend to use that style without even knowing it. I enjoyed the abstract painting class as I learned about different abstract styles and experimented with all of them. l was surprised that famous abstract artists, including Picasso, started out painting traditionally and then moved on to express revolutionary vision and imagination in abstract art.

I do not have a particular theme for painting. I like painting animals, landscapes, monuments, people, portraits, still-life, and I paint with acrylic and oil paints mostly, but I am open to all kinds of techniques. I continue to paint in between my other projects of writing, piano playing, lessons in Chinese, yoga, and bike riding, but most importantly spending time with my children. When I look back at my first experiences with painting in retirement, I am happy that I took different classes at the community learning center, which provided me with the necessary information and gave me confidence. I loved the classes as I developed friendship with the art teachers and the participants by receiving feedback, support, and encouragement for my work. Nowadays, with access to the internet and social media it is easy to find information on how to draw and paint. I also attended painting classes offered by Painting with a Twist, a program with classes which provide step-by-step instruction on how to complete a painting in a short time. I will never forget meeting a woman at the Dallas airport, who shared with me how she had been depressed since she retired and how she was thinking of going back to work. I asked her if she had any hobbies, such as painting. Her eyes lit up and she told me that she would love to paint and that she had even bought a canvas, paints, and brushes, but did not know how to start. I shared with her my experience, and I could see from the expression on her face that she was happy to find a solution to her problem. And I felt good that I helped a woman who was depressed after retirement.

I have heard that art heals the soul, and I believe it. It allows me to see and understand the world in a different way, as my mind transcends various spheres of consciousness to reach what I desire and intent to project in a painting. It has made me more observant and has boosted my self-esteem for being able to create paintings which speak about my feelings.

Creating art has tremendous benefits. It improves one's ability to solve problems; it improves memory and concentration, develops creativity, and lowers stress, because it creates calmness. In addition to making art, I thoroughly enjoy viewing it. My husband and I share a passion for art and have visited some of the most renowned art museums in the world. Museums contribute to my emotional health and stability, as my mood is uplifted just by walking in them. I love to stroll in a museum and get immersed in the lives of famous artists by the messages of their beautiful paintings with scenes of nature, people, portraits, and abstract visions. I will never forget my daughter at the Institute of Art in Chicago, running from painting to painting with a big smile, taking photos of most paintings with the information next to them. I was pleasantly surprised and very happy to watch her having so much fun.

Walking in art museums is also a great exercise that you hardly notice, since your attention is fixed on the art works.

The next chapter describes my visits to famous museums throughout the world. I did not compare my remarks to those of art critics. My comments are spontaneous, with reactions and feelings at the time of viewing the paintings.

CHAPTER 10
The Enchanting World Of Art Museums

PRADO MUSEUM - MADRID, SPAIN

Mitt and I visited the Prado Museum in Madrid in the spring of 2012. This was my first visit to the city, and I wanted to see the displays of world class art at the famous Prado Museum. Since our sightseeing time was limited to two days, we spent the first morning at the museum, admiring remarkable paintings by Goya, Velasquez, El Greco, Rubens, and Bosch.

I particularly remember Goya's *La Maja Desnuda* in two versions—naked and dressed. Nudity was not acceptable according to Catholicism in the late 1700s in Madrid, and every time a clergyman was expected at his house, Goya would put the painting of the dressed lady over the nude one. According to the guide who told us this story, Goya escaped prosecution by citing names of other artists with paintings of nudity who were liked by the church.

Diego Velasquez's *Las Meninas*, dating from mid-1600s, is known to be as captivating as the *Mona Lisa* in Louvre. The painting is a scene in the main chamber of the Royal Alcazar fortress near the Royal Palace. It has been described as a snapshot of people from the Spanish court. Some look in different directions, while others interact with each other. Velasquez included himself in the back of the scene, painting on a big canvas. I stood in front of the painting for a while, examining in detail the entire composition, the pose and position of each personality, the expression of their faces, their clothing, and the colors. I particularly enjoyed the painting because of the liveliness and spontaneity of the scene.

Bosch's *Garden of Earthly Delights*, painted around late 1400s and early 1500s, is phenomenal. It is done on three panels, depicting, from left to right, Paradise, with unique figures and machines; a garden with a lake in the middle, populated with fantasy creatures and people; and Hell, painted in dark colors with demons and burning cities. Bosch seemed to have wanted to share his understanding of sin, morality, and punishment.

El Greco's *The Trinity* was, for me, impressive, not only because of its religious character, but the dramatic illustration of the figures, including Jesus Christ ascending into Heaven.

Ruben's *Garden of Love*, a tribute to his second wife, is a happy scene of rich people, which is clear from their clothing, who are gathered in a park, with relaxed demeanors depicted in their postures and facial expressions. Here again I paused for a while, studying the very skillful scene's composition, communicating the exactness of the personalities and their interaction.

Rembrandt's portraits and Vermeer's paintings of mostly women in Netherland's homes in the 1600s were also featured in the museum.

THYSSEN AND REINA MUSEUMS –
MADRID, SPAIN

Mitt, being an avid art lover, took me to Thyssen and Reina museums. I remember Dali's surrealist painting in Reina Sofia Museum, *The Great Masturbator*, that looked like a fat cow, with woman's face in profile and squiggly lines completing the body of an animal with a funnel under the neck of the woman, which looked like it might be her vagina.

Thyssen Museum is astonishing, with paintings by Van Gogh, Gauguin, Cezanne, Picasso, Dali. Van Gogh's painting *Les Vessenots in Auvers* stood out with its fabulous landscape. In this painting Van Gogh shows us village houses amid meadows below a hill painted with bold strokes of green and yellow, so typical of Van Gogh, and perhaps showing his nervous state of mind before his suicide.

Paul Gauguin introduced me to Tahiti, with exotic paintings of tropical jungles and brown, darkhaired women bursting with life. It is this colorful, lively presentation of the Pacific Islands, which led me to visiting them later, and discovering their natural beauty with the crystal blue, turquoise, aquamarine, royal-blue interchanging watercolors, and the colorful, green vegetation in the jungles.

Paul Cezanne's style of loose, semi-abstract painting, which is representational enough to let you know what the painting is about, is a style I like and hope to adopt eventually for my paintings. *The Sainte Victoire Mountain* is a perfect illustration of a beautiful region, with definite shapes of trees, fields, and houses with a mountain in the back, which are abstract but recognizable.

Here I learned about Picasso's cubism, where paintings again are recognizable but not in a representational way.

Dali's surrealism is evident from his painting *Pierrot with a Guitar*, where there is a face, but it is difficult to distinguish the guitar and the body of the guitar player.

RIJKSMUSEUM – AMSTERDAM, THE NETHERLANDS

The Rijksmuseum houses memorable paintings by Rembrandt, Vermeer, Van Gogh, and Hendick Avercamp.

I can close my eyes and see Vermeer's *The Milkmaid*, which shows a girl pouring milk. Rembrandt's *Night Watch* is a sketch of thirty-four people, mostly in a shadow, all in motion, with three light visible personalities in its foreground, a man dressed in black with red sash, another in yellow with white sash, and a woman carrying a chicken. This painting I remember because of its size and the fact that it is extremely vivid.

Hendrick Avercamp's *Winter Landscape* is similar in style to Bosch and Brugel paintings.

ROYAL MUSEUM OF FINE ART –
BRUSSELS, BELGIUM

We visited Brussels for one day only and barely had a few hours to spend at the Royal Museum. I did not expect to see six museums connected with the Royal museums, with over twenty thousand works of art. We practically raced through the museum, so I will share a couple of paintings that impressed me the most.

The Fall of Rebel Angels by Bruegel, a renaissance artist, is a very dynamic painting of Lucifer falling with his angels as described in Revelation 12 of the New Testament. I recognized the influence from Bosch in the distorted, ugly, exaggerated, half-human figures.

The Census of Bethlehem also by Bruegel is easy to recall. It is a winter religious scene at sundown, with small figures engaged in daily activities which are difficult to discern. Joseph and Mary are on a donkey on the left side of the painting, and there is a cart with large wheels in the center. I picked to describe Bruegel's religious paintings because they are extraordinary artistic presentations.

PERGAMON MUSEUM BERLIN

At the museums in Berlin, I felt like I was in Greece. They are a major attraction in the center of the city. We visited first the Pergamon Museum. Its name derives from its main attraction, which is the altar of the Greek god Zeus, built as a testimony of the victory of civilization over barbarity. I am primarily interested in paintings, but this museum had a spectacular collection of sculptures, pottery, and jewelry from ancient Greek and Roman times, housed in its Antiquity wing. One of the most interesting pieces is a huge sculpture from the 2nd century BC, representing the struggle of the gods and the giants from Roman antiquity. I remember the museums art collections of architectural works, such as the colorful Ishtar gate and the Market gates.

NEUES MUSEUM – BERLIN

Neues Museum is another representation of Greek's mythology, with the bust of Queen Nefertiti and other objects from that era.

BODE MUSEUM – BERLIN

At the Bode Museum I viewed a collection of sculptures and art, coins, and crafts from the Byzantine Empire.

ALTES MUSEUM – BERLIN

Built in the early 1800s, the Bode Museum houses vases, bronzes, jewelry, and a Green handblown vase stand with black squiggly lines and blue spots by them.

MUNICH – ALTE AND NEUE PINAKOTHEK

ALTE PINAKOTHEK

The paintings in this Alte Pinakothek are from 14th through the 18th century. Two that I remember from our visit are *The Fall of the Damned* and *The Rape of the Daughters* by Rubens. *The Fall of the Damned* depicts the entangled bodies of damned people thrown into abyss by Saint Michael and angels, and *The Rape of the Daughters* is a very dramatic scene of two naked women, one grabbed by a man and another with a man behind her, along with two horses with their front hoofs in the air and a child.

NEUE PINAKOTHEK

As its name suggests, the Neue Pinakotek Museum houses art from a newer-age, 18th and19th centuries. This museum displays art works of prominent artists: *Sunflowers*, Van Gogh; *Water Lilies*, Monet; *The White Dress*, Klimt. I had seen photographs of these paintings in books, and I recognized the style of each artist—Van Gogh with nervous strokes, Monet with delicate colorful images of nature, and Klimt's paintings of standing women. They are all descriptive of the artist's feelings and mood. And this is a skill that I would like to acquire for my paintings as I still try to find my style by looking at different artists and their paintings.

ORSAY MUSEUM – PARIS

Both Mitt and I have been to the Louvre, so when we went to Paris, we decided to visit a different museum, the Orsay. This museum boasts paintings by famous artists. I immediately recognized Monet's *Water Llilies* in their delicate and realistic form, but still in a very loose presentation. I recognized the painting as soon as I saw it because of the unique presentation of the flowers.

Renoir's distinctive style is at once detected in his painting *Ball at the Moulin de la Galette,* which portrays content, happy faces of rich people evident from their clothing and the luxury of their surroundings. I stopped at this painting, as it is an expression of people having a great time dancing, sitting, and chatting around a table with drinks. Observing the painting immediately put me in a good mood, which seemed to be the intent of the artist.

Degas is also easily recognizable with his exquisite paintings of ballet dancers. Here it was in front of my eyes, *The Dance Class,* a beautiful painting of girls in pointe shoes (one is walking forward). They are in ballet dancer dresses, gathered around their teacher, an elderly man, leaning on a cane. The painting depicts intense emotion and joy expressed on the girls' faces.

Klimt also owned a peculiar and distinguishable style, and his painting *Rose Bushes Under the Trees* grabs your attention with its dotted apples, roses, bushes, trees, and grass. I recognized him from the rose bushes, which were painted in a shape of a woman. The predominant colors of white, red, green, and yellow are not bold, but rather soft, instilling peace and tranquility by the harmony in nature.

Manet's *Olympia* is a very realistic painting of a prostitute, lying naked in bed, staring directly at you with a bold, arrogant look, as if saying "What, I am not ashamed of what I do for a living." A colored lady nearby is delivering flowers to her with a look that can be interpreted as concerned, or maybe disappointed.

MUSEUM OF FINE ART – LYON

Arriving in Lyon on a short visit we headed to what is known to be one of the largest museums in France and Europe. It was easy for us to access this 17th-century building situated in the center of the city. My expectations of a delightful afternoon were met, as I felt privileged to view works of the best known artists on earth, such as Picasso, Perugin, Monet, Veronese, Rubens, Manet, Matisse, Gauguin.

In my quest to develop my painting skills and find a style of my own, I have been attracted to abstract art with bold colors in free and loose painting, but at the same time with identifiable figures and landscapes. I found Vlaminck paintings helpful for my taste as I could tell what the paintings are about as in *Houses at Chateaux*. There are houses in the background with trees and landscape in the front, but the presentation was what impressed me as I studied each of his strokes with bold, different colors, which were somewhat realistic for the trees, the ground, and the house. The sky was the closest to being real with various blue colors, a touch of purple and white clouds. I was truly amazed by the vibrant and happy feeling that this painting evoked in me.

Another artist whose work grabbed my attention was Modigliani. His paintings were different in style, since he painted only people, mostly portraits. I could not stop wondering why the female figures were so exaggerated, with long necks, asymmetric facial features, and unattractive bodies like the painting of *Jeanne Hebuterne*, a woman with a long nose, and a head out of proportion relative to her body. *The Girl in a Sailor Blouse* is similar with her long neck, and head way above the body. You would think that such paintings cause confusion, but they bring tranquility because of the soft expression on the women's faces. And I suppose the unique style has helped to make the work recognizable and remembered.

Next, we looked at Miro's paintings, which struck me as busy and abstract with figures, images, or objects in bold colors and shapes. I remembered from my readings that abstract art is an expression of colors and shapes and staring at Miro's paintings I could tell that he had planned the composition.

In Lyon's Museum I discovered an unforgettable Monet's painting, different from the joyous garden party gatherings, a painting called *La Tamise a Charing Cross* (Charing Cross Bridge). Hearing the story of the artist's thirty-seven paintings of the bridge in London at different times, I immediately recognized the one with a fog enveloping the scene with hardly distinguishable buildings in the back. For me this obscurity created feelings of mysticism, of search for the unknown. The use of the gentle blue, white, green, and yellow colors made me feel tranquil and calm.

From the Matisse collection, several paintings of women stand out, one of a woman in a white dress and another in a blue dress. Being new to painting I realized that I could partially adopt Matisse style of omitting details in the shape of hands or facial features. The backgrounds also are not exact, although they show the locations and the objects. The bright colors are well coordinated, evoking a feeling of happiness. Another painting I liked was Picasso's *Woman Sitting on the Beach*. There are some distinguishable parts of a naked woman's body, not in the right places, and extremely exaggerated. I can't say that I find beauty in this painting, but it is clearly sensational and unforgettable.

COPENHAGEN – GLYPTOTEK

The walk from the pier where the cruise ship docked along the canal and through the pedestrian part of town to the Glyptotek Museum was very enjoyable. The name of the museum comes from the Greek words of carve and storing place. I knew from a reading that the contents of the museum were a private collection. It was mostly a sculpture museum, but I was more attracted to the paintings of the famous artists, Monet, Pissarro, Renoir, Degas, Cezanne, and Van Gogh.

I particularly liked Cezanne's still-life paintings of apples in dishes and a folded cloth. The way he paints light and darkness is unique as it adds to the authenticity of the scene.

The painting of nude women bathing in nature is vivid, with figures in various positions, standing and looking forward, sitting and in profile. It is painted in soft light, blending colors of beige, green, and greyish blue; nature is painted very loosely, as the artist used different shades of green and grey to let us know that this is an outdoor scene. This painting produced in me a sensation of naturalness and simplicity because of the way life should be lived, without the shame of the nude body. Even the still-life painting had a clear display of how an eye can catch the different nuances of the painted objects.

Here I also recognized Degas ballet dancers in different poses and progress toward becoming prima ballet dancers. I could tell that Degas was fascinated by ballet movements and by the girls performing it. I always admired the ballet, especially the performance of *Swan Lake*, which we saw in St. Petersburg. These paintings brought back happy memories from our travels. Here I would like to add that a scene of a painting can affect us by triggering emotions related to experiences from the past.

Pissarro's *Pont Neuf* with statue of Henry IV has a style that I find close to Cezanne's; the images and the entire scene are loosely painted, but I could still tell that there was a bridge with people walking on it and trees in front of the buildings across. The difference that I found between the two artists is that Cezanne's paintings have bright, bold colors, while Pissarro's paintings are in darker colors. My interpretation is that the choice of colors reflects the artist's disposition or personality.

PORTUGAL – GULBENKIAN MUSEUM

We knew what to expect to see at the Gulbenkian Museum from the brochures at the hotel. The museum houses an incredibly valuable art collection that was owned by a single individual, Calouste Sarkis Gulbenkian, an Armenian oil magnate and philanthropist who lived in Lisbon from 1942 until his death in 1955. We did not spend much time in the museum's Greco-Roman section, but concentrated on viewing European art. We skimmed through halls with beautiful objects of different ages and headed to the art exhibits. I remember paintings that depicted real experiences and people, such as *The Boy Blowing Bubbles* by Manet, a painting of the illegitimate son of his future wife. What struck me was that the boy was not young to be entertained by blowing bubbles, which suggested the brevity of life. Renoir's style of painting women's faces stands out in the *Portrait of Madame Claude Monet*. I remember an interesting work by a painter I had not heard of, Sir Edward Burne-Jones's *The Mirror of Venus*, which shows Venus standing in a pale blue dress, surrounded by her maids dressed in beautiful orange-brown dresses, leaning over to look at their reflections in the water in front of them. What attracted me to view this painting was the beauty of the women, and the expression of sadness in their faces, suggesting that something was missing in their lives. The surroundings were rocky, and the hills were arid, with no greenery or vegetation. It's like placing beauty in a very depressing environment.

A more lighthearted painting was Monet's *Woman with a Parasol* of Madame Monet and her son. This scene is serene and peaceful with a portrayal of green meadows and blue skies, with scattered clouds in wavy shapes.

LONDON – THE NATIONAL GALLERY

Located at Trafalgar Square, London's National Gallery was easy access since our hotel was just around the corner from it. We were pleasantly surprised to find out that entrance was free. The National Gallery in London is a majestic building dominating Trafalgar Square. For me it had a special meaning not only because of its well-known reputation, but because I could finally visit it after dreaming about it since my high school years. The following paintings offer a glimpse of the exhibits in London's National Gallery.

Van Gogh's *Sunflowers* are in a vase, since his original paintings had the sunflowers laying down. It's a painting in Van Gogh style; the vase is asymmetric, and the flowers are in disarray, perhaps describing the state of the painter. Predominant yellow shapes fill in the entire painting. The sunflowers, broken by a bit of green color, did not evoke happy feelings in me, as it is not a lively scene, not what one might expect when viewing sunflowers in nature.

Monet's famous painting of water lilies was here. They can be spotted from a distance as Monet's impressionist style of painting lilies is distinguishable with the use of dots.

Da Vinci's *Virgin on the Rocks* is notorious for the serene divine scene created of a virgin young woman surrounded by three small children in an ambiguous setting of rocks with water in the background. I discovered that Da Vinci painted several versions of this same painting, changing some details, which makes me think that all these masters worked on one painting for a while to present the same scene in different lights. What is peculiar about this scene is that it produces a calming effect.

Velazquez's *Rokeby Venus* is also a serene scene of a nude woman, Venus lying on her side, with a small naked child angel on his knees holding a mirror up to her face. The setting is in a luxurious environment, as the bedding and the drapes suggest affluence. The painting is attractive and made me think of the hidden beauty of nature in the face of Venus.

The most viewed painting could be spotted from a distance, Jan Van Eyck's *The Arnolfini Portrait*. The crowd around it was staring at the painting of a pregnant young woman in a green dress with one hand on her belly and a man clothed in black with black felt hat holding her other hand. He also seemed to be making the sign of a cross. The background was in a darker colored bedroom in contrast to the brightness in the woman's painting. I interpreted the scene as a couple expecting a child. At first, I thought the man was a clergy because of his long dark gown and his signing with one of his hands. However, looking closer, it's obvious that his attire is not that of a priest. The dog at their feet adds to the family scene in the bedroom.

There is a lot more to see at the National Gallery, but the scope of this book is to provide only a flavor of what one could expect to see.

TATE MODERN GALLERY – LONDON

Tate Modern Gallery is worth seeing for its unique modern architecture. It resembles a pyramid at the base, but the sides are not equal, and the top is flat. The exhibits are of international contemporary modern art. Two artists whose work I enjoyed are Gilbert and George. Their paintings feature vivid colors, and abstract figures.

THE VICTORIA AND ALBERT MUSEUM – LONDON

Victoria and Albert Museum is an attractive architectural building, with a beautiful garden that has elliptical water feature, making it very refreshing in the summer months. Art objects thousands of years old, including ceramics, silver, medieval objects, sculpture, and costumes fill a vast area of the museum. It has a charming atmosphere, providing an enchanting walk among artifacts of ancient cultures.

BRITISH MUSEUM

The museum is a marvelous collection of art objects from centuries ago. As in other European museums, a vast number of exhibits are from other countries, including thousands of sculptures from Nigeria. The building itself is impressive, reminiscent of Greek architecture, with columns and sculptures at the entrance depicting the progress of civilization. We followed the map which we received at the entrance and started our tour with the Egyptian galleries, where I saw the Rosetta Stone, with its ancient Egyptian hieroglyphs, believed to unveil the mystic Egyptian history and beliefs in afterlife. The Greek Sophilos vase from around 600 BC is an impressive bowl for wine, decorated with scenes from Greek mythology. The Parthenon Sculptures are from a temple dedicated to goddess Athena, the patron deity of Athens. The bust of Ramesses the Great is worth mentioning as it belonged to an Egyptian pharaoh, who reigned in the 1200s. The figure is enormous, and it weighs tons of kilos.

A day at this museum is like a walk into the land of fairy tales from Greek and Egyptian mythologies. I am sharing a small part of what the museum offers to provide a taste of what one could expect to see and experience.

CHICAGO – INSTITUTE OF ART

What made the visit to this museum special and unforgettable was because my daughter Vanesa joined me, and it was connected to my participation in the Bulgarian Cultural Center Book Bazar, at which I was going to present my book, *New Beginnings: From Behind the Iron Curtain to America*. This visit was enjoyable also, because we met a Bulgarian lady who spent the entire day with us showing us the city and the art institute. It was a day full of pleasant emotions and experiences.

Considering the time limits, we headed to the exhibits, which we all preferred, the ones of impressionism and modern art. I had seen the exhibits before with Mitt, while visiting his grandsons at Chicago University, but this time was different. I felt such a joy watching my daughter hurry from one painting to another, examining each one carefully for composition, colors, meaning, depth, reading about the artists, taking photos, and turning to me with a smile.

"Surprised you, didn't I," she said jokingly, as she knew that I did not expect her to be so much interested in art.

"You sure did," I responded, smiling back at her. I love the art institute, but what I enjoyed the most was seeing my daughter having so much fun.

Both my daughter and I admired the following paintings: Pierre Bonnard – *Earthly Paradise* and *The Seine at Vernonnet* are both scenes in nature done in vivid, realistic colors, and in a style both impressionism and abstract.

Piet Mondrain's *Farm near Duivendrecht* is an attention-grabbing painting, with striking colors portraying a farm building and bare trees reflected in the water of a pond or stream painted in fall colors of different nuances of violet, blue, yellow for the sky, grey for the walls of the farm that are contrasted with the darker colors of the farm's roof and trees.

Grant Wood's famous *American Gothic* is a portrait of an austere-looking man and a woman standing in front of a house in a style known as carpenter gothic. The man has a pitchfork in his hand, and the houseplants behind the woman are thought by some to symbolize the genders in the household.

Archibald J. Motley Jr.'s *Nightlife*, a painting of a Chicago painter, is a very vivid, dynamic portrayal of a night scene in a bar with people dancing, sitting, and drinking at tables and at the bar. The bartender is reaching out for bottles in the background. The images are skillfully presented in vibrant colors to grab attention.

Edward Hopper's *Nighthawks* tells a story. A woman and a man are at a counter of a café, conversing with the waiter. Another man is sitting nearby with his back to the viewer. The woman seems to be engaged in a conversation, as one of her arms is lifted as if to gesticulate. The man next to her has a long face, listening, and the waiter is looking at the woman, appearing to be very interested in what she is saying and responding to her. The man sitting nearby had his head tilted as if eavesdropping. The dark-blue color behind the window in the background suggests that it is a night scene. It is my understanding that the name of the painting, *Night-hawks* implies that these people are night people. I like it because of the liveliness of the scene and the choice of colors.

Salvador Dali's *Inventions of the Monsters* is a sinister surrealist painting of monster images of the world, as Dali saw it during the Spanish Civil War. Horrific images surround a man and a woman sitting at a table, their faces close to each other, looking at objects on the table.

Claude Monet's *Cliff Walk at Pourville* and *Etretat: The Beach and the Falaise d'Amont* are two sea scenes that are similar in style, and both exhibit Monet's skillful choice of colors and shadowing.

PUSHKIN ART MUSEUM – MOSCOW

The Pushkin Art Museum has over seven hundred thousand works of art and consists of three buildings. The museum opened its doors for the first time in 1912. I visited the Pushkin Museum in 1995, while working for the International Monetary Fund on a project for tax reforms. I and the other foreign advisers were extremely excited to be able to view the galleries of world-famous paintings. On the day of our visit there was a new exhibit of paintings that had been seized and hidden by the Germans in the Second World War and taken back by the Russians at the end of the war. The line was incredibly long, winding around the building, with an estimate wait of three to four hours in below-twenty-degree temperatures. My colleagues looked at me with questionable expressions, and here is when my knowledge of Russian came handy. We went to the side of the building where the doors were guarded by a couple of guys in uniforms. I explained to them that my colleagues and I worked at the Ministry of Finance and that we had limited time, because of the nature of our work. I asked them if they could let us in, and they did. We were all ecstatic, as this was a historical event and an opportunity to see these treasured paintings.

Some of the most known art masterpieces are the Cranach paintings. *Adam and Eve* is a painting of a biblical scene with docile animals and Adam, who appears hesitant to take the bitten apple by Eve. There were several paintings by Vincent Van Gogh. *The Red Vineyard* is a painting typical of Van Gogh's style, with images and figures of bent women working in the field, and a man in a cart in the background. The landscape, with the field, the sky, distant houses, water, are painted with Van Gogh's usual definite strokes and colors for harvesting the crops with the women painted in blue to be identified in the field. Degas' *Blue Dancers* is one of the famous Degas ballerinas' paintings showing the girls in blue outfits performing a ballet with feminine, expressive movements.

Henri Matisse's painting *La Fenetre a Tanger* is a painting of a landscape viewed through a window. Done predominantly in different shades of blue, it is a cross between abstract and representational art, as the houses are identifiable, but the rest is left to imagination.

The Pushkin Museum has some of Monet's water lilies that show his unique ability of painting lilies. The colors, predominantly green, are of different nuances to separate the vegetation from the willow and other trees, bushes, and the floating white and blue lilies among green leaves.

The Priams Treasure exhibit is remarkable, as it is a collection of golden objects, bowls, and vessels from ancient Troy. Ownership of these items is in a dispute between Turkey and Russia, since there were found in Anatolya, Turkey, formerly Troy.

Another valuable collection we saw at the Pushkin Museum is an exhibit of paintings, drawings, and ceramics by Picasso, including some of his early paintings, such as *Embrace*—a man embracing a young woman in a room with a bed and chair. It is a simple scene which intends to show the couple's emotions, as they embrace and kiss. The colors are simple, blue, white, and red, to emphasize the simplicity of love between two people. The museum also has several paintings by Picasso's later work.

In retrospect I can share that my favorite painters are Matisse, because of his realistic paintings in an abstract presentation; Picasso, because of his developing style from realistic to abstract, which is based mostly on shapes with bold colors. I also enjoy Renoir for his lively scenes, and Monet with the famous landscapes and water lilies.

CHAPTER 11
Travel—Medicine For The Body, Mind And Soul

Travel is an activity that impacts health with long lasting physical and spiritual effects. Following are examples of how travel plays a significant role in a person's life:

1. Travel is a mood enhancer that fights depression and anxiety and improves sleep. When I travel, I leave things behind and immerse myself in the new world around me. I recall how my heart jumped with joy during a trip to French Polynesia at the view of the open market in Papeete with its amazingly beautiful plants and flowers and a fish market with fish of different colors, shape, and size. And a visit to a black pearl farm will always cheer up a woman.

2. Travel to beautiful and remarkable beaches in the Caribbean, Mexico, South America helped my husband endure and combat severe chemo cancer treatments. What we did after every chemotherapy was travel to resorts in Mexico and even went on a trip to Rio de Janeiro. My secretary at the time told us that he had a similar cancer, and at one point was giving up when his friend had him watch a video from Hawaii, which revived him and gave him strength to fight the sickness.

3. Travel is better than solving crossword puzzles, because it stimulates the brain to memorize places and people. When I travel, I like to learn a few foreign words from the country that we visit. This practice is a good memory booster as it makes you remember words for communication.

4. Travel is one of the best exercise programs. When I travel, I am constantly on the move. I walk from dawn till sunset, I hike, run, swim,

snorkel, and bike ride, depending on the location. A busy travel schedule keeps me in good shape and has a positive effect on my mind. Being outdoors I connect with nature on the beaches, mountain slopes, and safaris. Such activities are great factors for combating depression, anxiety, or nervousness.

5. Travel boosts confidence when you discover that you can get around well in a strange place. For example, finding the right metro line on the Tokyo metro is quite an accomplishment.

6. Travel is a source of energy, because a new environment stimulates the brain, makes you feel refreshed and ready to face daily life when you return home.

7. Travel enhances communication skills because communication is necessary to get around, understand information, and respond when needed. As a language lover, I enjoy practicing my speaking skills in French, Spanish, and recently Chinese. I loved chatting with a French lady on the Glass train in Switzerland, and finding out that relationships between parents and grown-up children are the same all over the world.

8. Travel enhances one's ability to evaluate situations and communicate with people. You may find yourself gesturing when trying to explain or ask a question. Booking a room in the wrong place, as I did in Marrakesh, might not be pleasant, but you learn to adjust and make the best of the situation. The hotel was in a primary sightseeing location and that was a big plus.

9. Travel enriches your knowledge in a way that reading a textbook cannot. You get firsthand knowledge of the history, geography, economic structure, infrastructure, school systems, and culture of the people who live in the places you visit. I was surprised to learn how in Togo, Africa, the school system and the good conditions of the roads were established during the German colonization.

10. Travel helps with the development of cognitive skills because it requires flexibility, organization, rapid planning, decision making,

which you will read about in this book, especially in the chapter of travel with Eurail in Europe.

11. It allows you to rediscover yourself and to get out of your comfort zone, as I did when I started to snorkel and felt a rush being surrounded by beautiful fish of all colors or when seeing a stingray and swimming beside a sea turtle.

12. Travel makes you appreciative of the things you have, like running water and electricity. It makes you aware of the liberties you have. For example, in China there is no Google, and we were relieved to know that at least we could use email. And there was no running water and electricity in a fishing village in Africa.

13. Travel makes you more creative at work, because after being exposed to new ideas and concepts you may take a different approach to problem solving or decision making. Retired people as well will improve their ability to handle tasks, as travel enlivens and boosts energy for people of all ages.

14. You become aware of the daily use of all your senses, like the smell of the sea, the forests, the flowers, the view of diverse scenes, the touch of sand under your feet, and the taste of food that leaves memories of certain places. The sounds of the birds and the music of places have the same effect. I will always remember the bird from the Maldives that makes a distinctive sound.

Travel is an important stimulant in life that is overlooked by a lot of people, perhaps because they are afraid to venture into unknown environments with foreign languages. It also could be apathy, lack of interest, or laziness that keep people in their neighborhood. The fact that in certain places world geography is not taught enough has deprived young people of this thirst for adventure and knowledge of the world. My curiosity about travel was aroused as a child growing up in Bulgaria when I read and studied geography. But that was during a communist regime, and what I saw were mostly documentaries of African tribes. Later, in my high school years, I was able to see photos of London and other cities in England shown by my English teacher and brought by students who could travel abroad. Back in those years I had the burning desire to travel, but the borders were closed for the common Bulgarian people, and I remained with my dream that one day I would be able to see these countries in the West or even be at the equator.

My dreams came true when I moved to America after escaping as a young girl from the communist regime in Bulgaria. The following chapters describe my travel in Europe, Africa, and Asia, where I viewed remarkable beautiful sceneries of mountains and seas, learned about ancient cultures, and visited historic sites, and monuments. The colorful presentation of folklore and cultural traditions and different intriguing ways of life in countries all over the world are invaluable lessons for diversity and the value of heritage.

CHAPTER 12
Travel Around the World

To make travel arrangements and get around the world is not as difficult as some might think. In most countries people speak English and are very glad and happy to help and give directions. Learning a few sentences is helpful when you travel in foreign countries. The French still cannot forget the hundred-year war with England, and they appreciate it if a foreigner tries to communicate in French rather than English. In China we asked the receptionist at the hotel to write in Chinese the name of the place we wanted to visit with directions how to get there. And people at the metro stations and in the streets were happy to help us. I also knew a few Chinese words.

With the travel chapters, I am sending you an invitation not only to enrich your life, but to feel more alive, energetic, and happy. I invite you to draw in your mind pictures from scenes of roaring oceans, waterfalls, and seas; peaceful villages tucked in gorgeous, majestic mountains; enchanting castles and temples; tropical forests and vegetation; and wild animals on safari in Africa. Feel the warmth from the smiling faces of people dressed in traditional colorful clothing and become enchanted by the beauty of the world! Take small trips at first to a neighboring country, and while staying at a resort, ask at the travel desk about excursions in the area. Rent a bike or a car with a driver and slowly expand the perimeter of the place that you are visiting. Learn from the internet about the most desirable things to do and visit while traveling based on the length of your stay. Your first choices can be countries where your native language is spoken.

We wanted to see most of Africa on both the east and west coasts, so we used the cruise line Oceania. The better lines are more expensive, but they give you a trip of your life by providing you with memorable, amazing, full-of-excitement, thrilling, and beyond-description experiences. For us, taking these trips was much more valuable than moving into a bigger house or buying a new car.

Cruises on a sail ship provide lifelong memories because they travel to smaller islands and offer views of incredible places. I have memories to last me a lifetime, from sailing to beautiful uninhabited islands in the Andaman Sea in Thailand to the twelve islands in the Caribbean, where I spent days in snorkeling and beach activities.

We saw in one month a substantial part of Europe by traveling with Eurail, the tickets for which we bought online in the States. It was summertime, and we traveled lightly, only with backpacks. Mitt oversaw the train reservations, which we took care of as soon as we arrived at the new place, and I booked all the hotels the night before traveling to a different city or country. I chose local three- to four-star hotels, which were economic, clean, attractive, and within walking distance of train stations and major attractions. Such trips require organization and good condition because of extensive walking and hiking like during our trip to Cinque Terre. As far as food, there are a lot of local inexpensive and attractive restaurants, such as the beer houses in Germany, the tapas in Spain, or the pasta and fresh seafood restaurants in Italy. We also had picnics with delicious local cheeses, prosciutto, salamis, fresh fruits, and wine. All sightseeing was preplanned, with recommendations from internet sites.

We also saw Spain by train without any prior reservations. We took a train from Madrid to Seville, and from Seville we traveled to numerous famous cities in the north all the way to San Sebastian.

Arranging private trips in Asia was simple as we booked flights and hotels on the internet for trips to Hong Kong, Japan, China, Thailand, Cambodia, Taiwan, Indonesia, Singapore, and Burma. All the hotels were local, centrally located, three to four stars, very clean, and comfortable. We chose the recommended sightseeing tours on double-decker buses to view all the sightseeing attractions and choose what sights to see in detail. We visited places suggested on the internet and the reception desks at hotels.

A lot of travel tips are given on YouTube Travel channels about places around the globe. We always watch such programs to learn important facts about the country we plan to visit. I like Rick Stevens' programs about travel to Europe. As a matter of fact, if you just type the name of a country, you will get detailed information depending on the length of your stay.

Most important is the feeling when we get back home from a trip. We feel rejuvenated, in an elevated mood, and always rediscovering the place where we live in comparison to what we saw and experienced in other cities and countries. Returning from my first visit to Thailand, I noticed how our town is not as colorful as the tropical cities of Bangkok and Chiang Mai. But what I appreciate is the comfort, cleanness, traffic, amenities, and order at home. I will never forget the Burmese and African people who live in huts and the African children who were happy to get candy and bottles of water. And they all looked so happy.

The following are descriptions of many of the trips we've taken, some considered to be the wonders of the world.

CHAPTER 13
Travel By Trains, Boats, And Planes

EUROPE

BULGARIA

Bulgaria is my homeland and is known in Europe as "Small Switzerland" because of its beautiful scenery. There are the Balkan Mountains stretching from east to west, dividing the country in North and South Bulgaria. The majestic Pirin and Rila Mountains, the latter with the highest peak in the Balkans of 2,925 meters, are close to the Greek border. The picturesque Rodopi Mountain is by the border with Turkey, and the Strandja Mountain is in southeast Bulgaria. The Vitosha Mountain is by the capital, Sofia, and Luylin is a smaller mountain, also by Sofia.

Growing up in Sofia, I developed my love for the mountains because it was customary to hike on Vitosha to the plateau and walk across to descend on the other side of the mountain. As a reward we used to stop at the chalet for a meal of kebapcheta (Bulgarian hamburger), fries, and a yogurt drink. I always wondered how difficult it would be to climb to the top Cherni Vrah (Black Peak), but I never attempted it until I was in my sixties, and Mitt, during one of our hikes on Vitosha, looked at me and said that we were going up rather than across the mountain. It was the steep side of the mountain to reach Cherni Vrah, but I did not object because I wanted to test myself and see if I could do it at my age. There was a lot of puffing and huffing during the climb, and at times I had to lower my hands to the ground not to lose my balance and fall backwards. We caught up with an Italian guy who asked us, in tears, if we knew of a way for him to get down on a less steep side. I managed to reach the top and stood proudly by the sign which showed height of 2,290 meters. One thing I remember is that because the altitude changed so fast I started to feel weak and dizzy. I did not realize that this was the fourth highest peak in Bulgaria after Musala. We descended from the less elevated part towards the Golden Bridges, and I immediately felt better. Golden Bridges, a phenomenon known as a rock river, is the favorite place for children. They love jumping from one huge rock to another, which is challenging at times. Adults like to sit on the rocks and have a picnic or lie down to sunbathe, enjoying the fresh mountain air and listening to the wind whistling in the trees.

Pirin Mountain is the region of the Pirin Macedonians, where I feel very comfortable because of my Macedonian heritage on my father's side. The songs and the music are close to those of Vardar Macedonia in former Yugoslavia and are very distinct from other parts of Bulgaria. I think they are very melodious and emotional.

On one hot summer morning while in Sofia, Bulgaria, Mitt suggested that we get out of the city to see some of the most picturesque places on Pirin Mountain and spend the weekend at a resort in the village Dobrinishte. We rented a car, and in a few hours arrived at a hotel with beautiful scenery of the Pirin Mountain, with slopes and hills which were lush and green in the summer months. After enjoying the day at the pool with mineral water, the spectacular views of the mountain, and the food at the Bulgarian restaurant, we planned for the next day to hike from Lodge Bezbog to Popovo Lake, the biggest lake in the Pirin Mountain. "Why is the name of the lodge Bezbog?" I asked Mitt.

"It is because the access to it is so difficult that even God cannot help you if you decide to climb up there."

"And what about the name of Lake Popovo?"

"There is a legend that a priest drowned in the lake, and only his clerical clothing was floating on the top, which gave the lake a shape resembling a clerical attire." One of the legends talks about the priest going to see the mean god Perun, who became enraged when he saw the priest with the holy water and dragged him in the lake, where he drowned, while his clerical clothing remained on the surface. I was intrigued to see this lake because it was considered a sacred place.

The open lift to the lodge offered the most spectacular mountain views. I deeply inhaled and filled my lungs with the intoxicating fresh air mixed with the smells of wildflowers and green trees and shrubs and then slowly exhaled with a smile. The Bezbog Lodge is an attractive building, with a roof which slopes down to the side, and has perfect rectangular windows and white shutters against the brown color of the wooden façade. The road from the lodge to the lake was just as described in all brochures, challenging at one steep spot with more elevation at times but not difficult. At least I did not need to use my hands this time as on Vitosha to keep my balance while climbing. Vendors from the village sold fresh fruit alongside the path, and when I asked one of them how long it would take us to get there, he responded: "Usually it's an hour-and-a-half hike, but for you, city folks, it will take three hours," which made us laugh. The sights kept changing with more breathtaking views of mountain beauty and in about an hour and a half we arrived at the lake. What a magnificent sight it was. The place was stunning, with tall mountain peaks reflecting in the water, and with wildflowers and bushes around the lake. We picked a spot by the water for our picnic and to spend the rest of the day admiring the beauty around us.

On another day we took a bus from Sofia to the resort Borovets, knowing that there was a lift from there to Lodge Musala. Borovets is a famous ski resort on Rila Mountain, visited primarily by Sofia residents as it is close to the capital. Mountain lodges tucked in forests of evergreen trees, views of the ski slopes, and the typical Bulgarian kitchen restaurants make this place extremely attractive. The lift was not working, so we decided to walk, not really knowing what to expect. It was a beautiful hike through meadows and forests, with birds chirping along the way. We climbed towards the top of the forest, where we believed that the lodge was. But then we discovered that we had to walk down and climb another high slope to reach the lodge. I remember stopping at a small wooden bridge with gorgeous flowers around it. I decided that this was a good spot for a break and for meditation among beautiful mountain flowers, listening to the creek from below. After hours of hiking, we reached a place from where we could see the lodge, but we needed to pass through a wet terrain and try to stay dry by hopping from one rock to another. At one spot I lost my balance and fell in the mud, which made me laugh. When we reached the lodge, we saw people in the front singing mountain songs, which put me in a festive mood. I could see Musala Peak, but after the long hike we were both too tired to think about climbing it. A little walk from the lodge took us to a lake where we found a suitable place for me to wash and dry my jeans, and then lie in the sun, enjoying the magnificent panorama and watching the rows of people climbing towards the peak and looking smaller and smaller like ants in the distance.

We have driven to the Pirin and Rila regions many times, visiting the well-known monastery Rila and the Baba Vanga site at the village Rupite in the Blagoevgrrad region. People used to spend days in tents, waiting to see the fortune teller Baba Vanga and hear her foretell their future. The mountainous part of the Rupite is a crater of the extinct volcano of Kozhuh Mountain and gives a mysterious look of Baba Vanga's house and church. Some people say that they feel energy when at the Rupite. For me it was a feeling of mysticism, of something unreal and magic. The night before you visited her, you had to put a sugar cube under your pillow. I saw her twice while I worked in Bulgaria as a tax advisor, and the only question I asked her was about the future of Bulgaria, for which she responded that my work would make a difference. This was all I wanted to hear.

Mitt and I took this trip again and relived the experience of being present in the surroundings of the majestic Rila and Pirin Mountains. On that day we visited the Rozen monastery. In existence since medieval times, it survived the rule of the Ottoman Empire and is the biggest monastery in the Pirin Mountains. Its location is in a very picturesque region, with rock formations resembling a pyramid and not far from the very famous wine-producing town Melnik. The place appears mysterious and is a source of spiritual strength for visitors. Near the monastery we visited the Yane Sandanski tomb of a great revolutionary fighter for the liberation of Macedonia. Significant for this gravesite is the inscription on it: *The slave fights for freedom, and the free man for perfection.* Staring at the tomb I thought of my Macedonian heritage and the time when at the age of nineteen I left communist Bulgaria in search of freedom.

The Rila Mountains, rival in beauty to Pirin, provide unforgettable memories of magnificent panorama and places of worship. Rila Monastery is a magnificent building where Eastern Orthodox religion is practiced. Consisting of a main church with beautiful domes and two side chapels, inside with three altars, gold-plated icons, and religious paintings, it is a remarkable site of historic, cultural, and architectural value. A walk up the hill takes you to a dark cave, leading to an exit through a hole. People who could get through are deemed to be without sins. I must admit that it was a little scary, stumbling inside the dark cave and then discovering that the hole was elevated, so I had to pull myself up to get out.

We continued our trip to the seven Rila lakes, well known for their magnificent beauty of colors blending in different shades of blue and green. It is a wonderful place to visit because of its serenity, charm, and mysticism. We drove to Sapareva Banya, from where we hopped on the two-seater lift for the lodge Seven Rila Lakes. The feeling was incredible when we flew over tall standing evergreen trees, meadows, shrubs, with a gorgeous view of the mountain around us and the city below. The lodge was at the foot of the first lake, the Fish Lake, but we wanted to go further up to see at least two more lakes. Getting off the lift, we followed a rocky path leading up a hill, and without even knowing it we reached a lake called Babrek. It was getting late, and we had to consider the working hours of the lift to return. We stood in amazement that there was snow around us. Naturally, we started a snowball fight. The panorama was captivating. The lakes were snugged between hills and peaks of different shapes and vegetation. As we headed back, I felt an incredible uplift of my mood and a feeling of happiness. Later I learned about a special divine New Year's celebration at the Rila Seven Lakes by a movement called The Universal Brotherhood, created by Peter Danov in 1897, which still existed. It is a teaching about the soul, the mind, and the heart. The main criteria are love, wisdom, truth, justice, and virtue. The purpose of the brotherhood is to help people discover the powers given them by God to establish a brotherly relationship between all nations on earth. They start celebrating at sunrise, with the performance of a special dance, *panevritmia,* which combines music, rhythm, movement, and thought. They say that when dancing panevritmiya, a person taps into the energies of nature and feels rejuvenated to extremity.

We planned to travel east and to reach the Rodopi Mountains, which provokes emotions with their majesty and beauty. We left Dobrinishe early in the morning, eager to see the Razlog Basin, where the three mountains— Pirin, Rila and Rodopi—meet. I was so happy to be at that place where the mountains display the distinct characteristics of their shapes, vegetation, and peaks. Rila is known to be high, Pirin beautiful, and the Rodopi Mountains, which spread all along the Turkish border, are gorgeous, with lush vegetation and forests of broadleaf and mixed trees. That day we were set to see Devil's Gorge. We drove on a narrow road that hardly allowed two cars to pass each other, so Mitt had to blow the horn every time we were close to a curve. But the panorama was divine. We drove between high cliffs alongside a river. At one spot I noticed people bathing, which looked so attractive on that hot, sunny day. There was a feeling of mysticism as we arrived at the entrance of the cave, which is considered mysterious because nobody knows what hides at the bottom of its river. Some people who came out of the cave were petrified, and others were afraid to go in.

At any rate, we had to see it. As I walked in, I had the feeling of getting into a devil's entry, about to be engulfed. A devil's head was carved in the walls as well as a figure of Orfei—a legendary prophet and musician of ancient Greek religion—and the image of Mary. There were the expected stalagmites and stalactites, and now that we entered a tunnel, we could hear the roaring water of the river. A huge hall appeared, and the roar became louder as we found out that there were eighteen waterfalls, with cascades underneath. The guide told us of the attempts of divers to get to the bottom and find out the course of the river to the point where it surfaces, but all of them perished. "There was an American who wanted to send a robot," the guide said, "but then he reevaluated the situation and did not want to lose his robot." From there on there was a climb of 301 steps on a narrow path leading to the surface, where the mysterious water appears again. It was already afternoon, so we headed to Pamporovo, a resort in the Rodopi Mountains, very well known for skiers, but just as attractive in the summer months. It was easy to find a room, and after checking in, we rushed out to explore the complex. There were numerous restaurants serving authentic Bulgarian food, and we could not resist but visit one and have a dish of roasted lamb meat.

Early next morning we took the lift to the recommended peak Snezanka, with an observation deck from a tower displaying marvelous scenes of mountain beauty. There were hills with century-old evergreen trees, and in the distance were the calm waters of the Smolyan Lake. To the north was the Balkan range, and to the west were the Pirin and Rila Mountains. From here we headed on foot to the Orpheus rock, a place where Orpheus received inspiration to play his lyre. Climbing on it, I felt an unexplained source of energy and happiness—something that Peruvian people were referring to when talking about Machu Picchu, but for me it was here where I experienced a powerful electrifying sensation. My eyes wandered from left to right, absorbing the beauty of the scene. I was in an awe of the view of aged evergreen trees disappearing slowly to a ravine of meadows, with the seven Smolyan lakes and more hills beyond it with gorgeous evergreen trees. From this enchanting place we headed to another spectacular Rodopi spot, the Wonderful Bridges. The best way to describe them is that they appear like amazing rock formations, with two bridges above openings in a rock surrounded in greenery. After this breath-taking place, we headed to the Black Sea.

When we arrived in Burgas, which is a major harbor on the Black Sea, I immediately felt the happiness of people who were on vacation. The streets were lively with men, women, and children who were in a hurry to get to the beach and spend a day of swimming, lying in the sun, playing in the sand, and having fun. We continued driving south and reached familiar places from both of our childhoods. Sozopol, which is the most ancient town on the Black Sea in Bulgaria, is a place that we remembered differently. Mitt did his military service here, and my memories were of spending precious times with my aunt at the beach. As we approached town, traffic became very congested, with crowds of pedestrians maneuvering among the vehicles. We managed to park and pick a place from which Mitt could see the barracks where he was stationed as an army doctor (the building was closed as it was not in use any longer). Alongside the promenade by the sea, we could see the restored watch tower and part of the ancient city walls. We headed to the old part of town, where I remembered how we took walks with my aunt, my cousin Nikolai, and his mom after a day in the sun. The town was as charming as I knew it from my childhood, with its ancient wooden houses and narrow cobblestone streets. And now it has a modern look, with outdoor restaurants, galleries, street vendors, and souvenir shops. We walked by the medieval ruins, deeply in thought of our different memories. In the past my aunt used to rent a room in one of those ancient homes with beautiful gardens, but now it was difficult to find a place without a reservation, so we headed further south.

As a child I had seen photos of the Ropotamo River, but now I had the opportunity to see it with the beautiful water lilies by Strandza Mountain, which was spectacular with its beech and oak trees and its evergreen bushes and plants of Mediterranean, Balkan, Central and Euro Asiatic regions. All the places where we stopped were full, even the very luxurious complexes, so we finally stopped in Varvara at a family-owned hotel by the road. It was a new building, and our room had a balcony with a view of the sea. The walk to the shore was about half an hour, but we didn't mind the little exercise after being in the car most of the day. We reached a restaurant with steep steps down to a small beach where we had the most delicious turbot fish and wine to celebrate the beauty of the evening. I fell on the way back, but that did not take away from the good mood, and I jumped in the pool as soon as we walked back to the hotel.

The next morning, we woke up rejuvenated from the fresh sea air, sun, and water, and hopped in the car to reach the border with Turkey. Driving along the coast was a delightful experience as we passed first at Tsarevo, a picturesque resort town in a cove with new and old architecture of villas and houses. The water looked so attractive that we pulled over at one of the last remaining uninhabited beaches, the Salistar Beach. Natural sand dunes and sand lilies on the beach made this place look like heaven. The couple of hours that we spent surrounded by the unspoiled beauty of this beach, sunbathing and swimming in the crystal-clear water, did wonders for us. Being close to nature in my homeland made me feel extremely happy. All my senses were awake as I admired the scenery, listened to the waves crashing at the beach and the noises of the seagulls, smelled the fresh sea air, tasted the sea water, and touched the fine sand. After a delicious fresh fish meal and a beer from the pavilion on the beach, we followed the road to view more attractive sea towns and villages.

Ahtopol is a place worth mentioning because of its ancient history and beauty. An old Thracian settlement, colonized by the Greeks around 440 BC, the place is a treasure of archeological findings. We stopped for a moment by the north gate of the medieval fortress, which was an amazing sight. Walking down the streets, surrounded by typical old Bulgarian houses was like walking back in time. Just a few kilometers south of the city were beautiful beaches at the estuary of the River Veleka. Following the picturesque road with the sea on the left and the Stranza Mountain on the right, we reached the village Rezovo, which was the last populated sea resort at the estuary of the Rezova River, the natural border with Turkey. Along the way we saw a couple of border patrol guys who just waved at us. What a difference from the communist era when nobody would dare come close to the border. I smiled back, and we proceeded to the place where the Bulgarian and Turkish flags were displayed. Across was a Turkish resort that for whatever reason looked empty.

There are additional breathtaking sights to visit in Bulgaria like the rocks of Belogradchik, the city of Tarnovo, which is an ancient capital of the country, the Cradle of Love—in the Balkan Mountains—The Hoof by the Kardzali dam and many more.

We both love city cultural life, and Sofia, the capital, offers spectacular theatrical and opera performances, visits to museums and galleries, and a variety of cultural events. It is easy to get around and view attractive sights, visit parks, and get a feeling about the rhythm of the city. If you visit Sofia, I recommend staying at Marriott at downtown's Nedelya Square with the ancient medieval church St. Nedelya. Walk straight ahead and you will reach the lively pedestrian boulevard, Vitosha, with outdoor restaurants and cafes, fashion outlets, flower shops, and bookstores, a boulevard always busy with crowds of people socializing over a cup of coffee or having a delicious meal. You will be staring at the peaks of the beautiful mountain Vitosha as you approach the park of the National Palace, a building holding cultural events with a restaurant on the top. I always check out schedules for interesting programs of famous concerts and shows. Take a walk behind the hotel and you will see archeological sites. Further to the right is the City Park, with the amazing architecture of the National Theatre and beautiful fountains in the front, the former King's Palace as an art museum, the grandiose cathedral Alexander Nevsky, and the building of the National Assembly with impressive architecture of neo-Renaissance style. Continuing down on Ruski Boulevard, you will see the impressive University building, opened since 1934. Across from it is a park, and if you venture further down, you will cross Eagle Bridge and walk in a park with a man-made lake and a restaurant. If you want to strike a conversation with a Bulgarian, the young people speak English, and you will learn all about the way they live. Most Europeans do not greet strangers in the street, but you will find that the personnel in the stores and the restaurants are very friendly. I recommend taking a cab to the famous Golden Bridges or the Aleko Lodge on Vitosha Mountain, from where you will have amazing views of the city, you will breathe the fresh mountain air and enjoy the scenery of flora, evergreen trees, and oak trees at the lower belt. For people interested in botany, there are five hundred different species of plants on the mountain, and for bird lovers, there are numerous species. There are reptiles and snakes, deer, wild boar, and wolves. I haven't come across any of the mentioned animals, but then I was told that wildlife animals stay away from the main paths. So, take a break from the hustle and bustle of the city to spend a splendid day in nature, and here people will greet you if you decide to take a little walk.

If you visit Plovdiv, the second biggest city in Bulgaria and the oldest in Europe, you need to head directly to Old Town, where you will see amazing old architectural and archeological wonders. Wear comfortable shoes and be ready to walk up a hill. Stop at the Amphitheater and check out for tickets if you have time as they give life performances, and then visit the Roman stadium. Walk on the cobblestone streets by numerous ancient houses, many of which are converted in museums, such as the Hinldliyan House of National, revival style with traditional Bulgarian architecture. The Balabanov House is recommended to be seen as a jewel of cultural beauty with its modern art paintings, sculptures, and mosaics. And don't miss Zlato Boyadziev Gallery and the Dimitar Kirov Exhibition. The artist Zlato Boyadziev is famous for the use of bright and distinct colors for painting old Plovdiv houses, landscapes with scenes of nature, and villagers dressed in folk attire. Dimitar Kirov is known in art circles for his abstract and modern paintings, which will satisfy the tastes of any admirer of abstract painting.

This concludes my stories about places in my homeland. I guarantee every visitor memorable times spent on majestic mountains, alongside the seacoast, or by amazing historical and archeological sites dating from 5000

BC. Most of all, you will enjoy Bulgarian hospitality and the healthy, delicious dishes; you will learn about folk dances and music that will grab your heart, and don't forget a souvenir of the famous Bulgarian rose oil.

TRAVEL IN EUROPE BY EURAIL

I remember being in my teens and daydreaming with my cousin Gabriela about traveling by train in Western Europe from one country to another and visiting all their capitals and well-known sights. We could visualize ourselves at train stations and imagined walking on streets leading from there to the center of towns with monuments, cathedrals, buildings, and parks. At the same time, we knew that travel to Western Europe from communist Bulgaria was impossible and forbidden. But sharing our thoughts out loud made these places alive. Gabi and I dreamed of traveling west all the way to England.

I was sixty-eight years old when Mitt suggested that we take that trip and visit the places I had dreamt of seeing as a teenager. "There is Eurail,

Nina, which is a pass to travel by train in Europe. We can travel in first class, and for a month we could stop wherever we want and stay for as long as we decide." My eyes lit up, as this was my wish from childhood. I had already been to a few countries while working as a US tax advisor to Bulgaria after the fall of the Berlin Wall, and prior to that as a teacher taking a group of my students to France. But a train backpacking trip was still on my mind and sounded very attractive.

"Let's plan it, then," I responded with enthusiasm.

The next couple of days we examined the map, researched how the Eurail pass worked, and designed an itinerary from Bulgaria to Serbia, Hungary, Austria, Germany, Switzerland, Netherlands, Belgium, France, Italy, and Greece. We outlined specific places that we considered "must see," and the rest we decided to play it by ear. We knew that we could not book any hotels as we had no idea when and where we were going to arrive from day to day. And armed with all the information that we gathered, we purchased Eurail tickets valid for twenty-eight countries in one month.

It was July 2017 when we arrived in Sofia, Bulgaria, and took the metro to Mitt's apartment. We were at a restaurant close to his place the night before the trip, eating local dishes with chitlings and *kachamak* (a corn-based meal like Italian polenta).

"I will not be carrying your backpack," Mitt said jokingly. He was referring to the fact that in the past, I considered backpacks to be just for hiking, and more for teenagers.

"I can carry it myself. Did you forget that I exercise at the gym and do weightlifting once a week?" I answered.

"Hmm" is all that he said, and we remained silent for the rest of the evening. We packed in the evening. I had learned to like backpacking since our trip to Peru and Ecuador the prior winter. It just required more organization. I was traveling in tennis shoes and a loose cotton sleeveless dress, which was comfortable for spending long days in train compartments. And I thought that if I forgot or needed something, I could always buy it.

Traveling to Belgrade brought memories of my student days when I took the train from Belgrade to Sofia almost weekly to see my family. There was no first class, so we were in the regular compartment, without air conditioning. Bulgarians do not like a draft, so there was an ongoing dispute about opening and closing windows. Ignoring them and the heat, I looked out the window, admiring the scenery. I enjoyed viewing the villages tucked below hills with cultivated fields in the front. The white painted houses suggested easy, relaxed country living. The extremely picturesque Sicevachka Klisura River Gorge formed by Nisava River was breathtaking.

It was a long trip that took nine hours to cover about two hundred miles. Sometimes it felt like it would be faster to walk. We arrived in Belgrade close to midnight and took a cab to our hotel, Marriott, which was surprisingly very reasonable in price and centrally located. We were exhausted, but we looked at each other and we knew that we would be going out. Skadarlija, the cobblestoned well-known street with restaurants serving typical delicious Serbian dishes and music going into the night, was in the back of the hotel. I remember being very tired as I walked towards the famous Tri Sheshira (three hats) restaurant. And there it was, an attractive one-story building with an open terrace in front. As I chewed slowly on the specialties of the night and listened to the life music of musicians serenating tables I remembered my student days. I used to visit with my friends from the university regularly Serbian *kafane* (pubs), and we had so much fun. Those were such carefree and happy times, I thought to myself. I loved to study, and life was so pleasant and enjoyable in the company of easygoing and open-hearted young people.

"It's getting late." Mitt brought me to reality, so we paid and returned to the hotel. We were catching a train to Budapest in the morning. After a few hours' sleep we checked out of the hotel and headed out into the street. We walked to Prince Mihailo monument in the Republic Square, the main square in the city, which was in front of the hotel. Prince Mihailo was a Serbian Prince in the 1800s and was known for his noble actions of favorable treaties with the Balkan countries. It was early morning, but there was already traffic, and people were rushing to get to places. The city was awake. We called a taxi and arrived at the train station early enough to have a delicious burek (cheese-filled fillo dough) for breakfast.

Soon we were on our way to Budapest. This train was very different. As it left the station it rapidly picked up speed. It was faster than the ride from Sofia to Belgrade, as it took about seven hours for a two-hundred mile trip, and we were in first class, with air conditioning. Looking out the window, I immediately recognized the Panchevo Bridge over the Danube and spotted the new Sava railway bridge in the distance over Sava, the biggest tributary of the Danube. Memories flooded about walking alongside the river as a student in Belgrade in the years 1968/'69. I visualized the beautiful paths with restaurants and coffee shops, and boats on a nice sunny day. I remembered the Belgrade fortress with the old citadel Kalimegdan, which overlooked the beautiful Danube and Sava riverbanks. The train continued north alongside scenes with cute small villages, fields of cultivated land, green meadows with lines of shrubs, bushes, and trees. We stayed in Budapest only half a day, and we had to make the most of it. We grabbed a cab to the most popular sight by the Danube, the Parliament. I could see it from a distance, a majestic building of neo-gothic architecture with a symmetrical façade of impressive towers, beautiful sculptures, and a central dome in the public square. We were there on time to observe the official ceremony of the changing of the guard. Behind Parliament was an equally marvelous sight, the Royal Buda Castle. It was so stunning that I remember tripping and almost falling trying to take a photo of it. Dating back to the 1200s, the majestic building provides an incredible picture. I was stunned by its amazing architecture and charm.

The night train to Germany reminded me of the overnight trips to the Black Sea with my aunt. I took the upper bunk bed in the sleeping car and soon dozed off in a sweet dream of colors and views of unknown places. A loud man's voice and noise outside the compartment woke me up. We were at the border with Austria. Mitt provided the necessary documents to the border control person, and we were on our way to Bavaria, Germany. Munich was a city I always wanted to visit, and here I was. Our hotel was a short distance from the railway station and occupied a couple of floors of an apartment building. We rushed outdoors as soon as we checked in and got settled into a clean and comfortable room. "Look, Nina, the name of this street is Einbahnstrase; remember it so we can find our way back." We both laughed because that word meant a one-way street. We turned around the corner and were pleasantly surprised to see that our hotel was just a couple of blocks away from the city center. We found ourselves at an amazing square called Marienplatz and in front of an impressive building, the New Town Hall, decorated with numerous statues and arches. And here on the building's tower was the famous Rathaus-Glockelspiel (clock), which gave animated performances of historical Bavarian events. It was dinner time, and we headed to a German's biergarten restaurant. I splurged on German sausages, while Mitt ordered a roasted pork knuckle, a very popular dish with meat that melts in your mouth. The side dishes of sauerkraut and specialty salads were tasty as well, and we toasted to our incredible voyage with a glass of the famous German beer. On the way back to the hotel we glanced at the cathedral of Gothic style with two towers, considered the landmark of Munich according to the lady at the reception desk.

The nearby castles were on our list to visit in the next days, as well as the impressive and tallest mountain peak, Zugspitze. The trip to the mountain top was unforgettable. We preferred to take a cogwheel train on a rack railway, which traveled inside the mountain, and took us to a platform called Zugspitplatt. From there we took a cable car. Reaching the top and standing on a beautiful roof terrace, we admired the panorama of alpine peaks in Germany, Austria, and Switzerland. Being on the border with Austria, we were entertained at the thought of visiting two countries at the same time, just by walking down a narrow passage. We were ready to return after a hot goulash soup.

"How do we get back?"

"Look down, there is the entrance to the train station," I pointed out, which made him relieved.

Following our sightseeing itinerary, we booked a tour to the two famous Bavarian castles, Linderhof and Neuschwanstein. They were both built by King Ludwig II who loved and adopted the artistic style of the French Sun King—Louis XIV. Linderhof seemed like little Versailles, with symbols of the sun throughout the castle. Similarity can also be seen in the size of the king's bedroom, which is the largest room in the castle. The castle was spacious, full of light, but also private and comfortable. In the dining room there was an area with a movable section on the floor, which was used to raise and lower a dining room table with meals from below, as Ludwig II was very reclusive and did not like company. It was the park and the gardens on the grounds of the castle that were stunning, a combination of formal gardens and English landscape. The remarkable Gilt fountain dominated the scenery with a twenty-five-meter high water jet. Neuschwanstein Castle looked like a fairy-tale building, which we saw as soon as we stepped off the bus. It is from the Romanticism era and has inspired the creation of Disney's Sleeping Beauty castle. We learned that the palace was built to honor Richard Wagner, since Ludwig II was an enthusiastic lover of art and music. The interior design is based on the legends of the Swan Knight from Robert Wagner operas. The castle was different from Linderdorf as it didn't have the feeling of intimacy and comfort.

A stop at a Bavarian village was unforgettable, with beautiful scenery of Bavarian houses with astounding wood carving and paintings on the outside walls with religious and fairy tale scenes. Of course, a stop for a strudel was in order, and here I tasted one of the most delicious strudel desserts.

My dream trip continued in the first-class, modern, and fast German train on our way to Switzerland. Zermatt was our destination since we wanted to reach the famous Matterhorn Mountain peak. The village looked like a postcard picture, surrounded by the highest peaks in the Swiss Alps with views of forests and ski slopes. A cobblestone street lined with chalets, cute hotels in Bavarian style, souvenir shops, and restaurants led us to our hotel, a mountain chalet. We were extremely happy to have a room on the last floor with a spectacular view of the Matterhorn summit.

We received information at the reception desk about traveling to the top and walked out to explore the place. We bought fruits, bread, cheese, and salami and had a picnic in a small park close to the hotel. Early next morning we left for the world-renowned peak. The trip was amazing as we took three cable cars from which we admired breathtaking, panoramic views over the Alps. Once on the top we headed to a viewing platform, but the day was cloudy, and we could not see the expected scenery of peaks and glaciers in Switzerland, France, and Italy. But we did get a glimpse of the spectacular Matterhorn Mountain. What was exceptionally stunning was the Glacier Palace, an ice cave with glittering ice sculpturers designed by talented artists. The most impressive was the panorama room with a sculptured mountain.

Switzerland is also famous for its glacier train, which we were eager to experience. Hopping on a train in Grindelwald, where we spent a night after Zermatt, we reached the station of the famous glacier train, which took us through the Alps to see amazing sceneries of lush green meadows, cute villages tucked in the valleys, or in the hills, and majestic mountain slopes with high snow-covered peaks. The train also passed by unforget-table places, like Interlaken tucked between two lakes with clear, turquoise waters with mountain ranges reflected in them. The scene was amazing, as the austerity of the mountains was soothed by the calming effect pro-jected by the green pastures. Since the train had tall glass windows, we could view the entire breathtaking scenery without having to change seats or hop back and forth across the aisle. Across from me was an elderly French woman who was taking a vacation by herself, with whom I ex-changed stories about our grown-up kids leaving the nest and having lives on their own. My French was not that rusty, I thought, as I could hold a conversation with her and understand her story.

Next stop on our tour was Amsterdam. Leaving the railway station, I immediately saw the canals that I read about as a teenager. And I had to see them all. We spotted a place where they offered tours on a boat, and that same day, after settling in a hotel, we headed to one of the piers. The ride was magnificent, taking us everywhere in the city with views of the Dutch Baroque houses from the 17th century. They were perched high, and appeared unassuming, with no richness or dramatic structures. The Jordan district was typical of the Amsterdam city life, with bikes stacked on bridges above the canal. A beautiful sight was the Herengracht Canal intersecting another canal with seven bridges. The rest of the day was dedicated to a very enjoyable walk in the Old Town. We reached Dam Square, with cobblestone streets and tall impressive historical buildings, and the magnificent Royal Palace. We walked alongside 9th Street, known for shopping, and we came upon WAAG (weigh house), a castle built in the 15th century. We passed by Anne Frank's house, but it was late in the day, and it was closed. Eager to see more, we followed the canal to the Red District, with sex shows and naked girls standing in the windows. Mitt suggested that we get some snacks, and I chose an ice cream. Sitting by the water we observed the pedestrians around us and the boats cruising up and down the canal. The city smelled of marijuana, and the square close to our hotel was trashed with garbage during the day, and meticulously cleaned at night. In the morning I woke up in bliss, feeling as I never felt before. I was melting in happiness, which was different from any other happy feeling that I had experienced before. Then I realized that the ice cream I had the night before probably had cannabis.

Our plan for the day was to visit the famous art Rijksmuseum, which housed eight hundred years of Dutch history and paintings of well-known artists as Rembrandt, Van Gogh, and Vermeer. I especially remember the famous painting of a milkmaid by Vermeer.

We were so close to Belgium that we planned a day trip to Brussels, where we walked by St. Michel Cathedral, listened to a delightful music performance, admired beautiful flowers in front of the Town Hall, and had Belgium waffles. We had picked places to see, so we visited the Grand Place, a tremendous square surrounded by historic buildings dating the 14th century, including the Town Hall, which is an impressive medieval building of Gothic style, decorated with statues representing local nobility. A statue of

St. Michael, the patron of the city, stands at the summit of the building's tower. We continued to the *Manneken Pis*, a statue of a boy peeing. I am not sure why it was designated as a tourist attraction, but it was cute. What really impressed us was the Royal Museum of Fine Arts, with paintings from the 15th to the 21st century, representing a tremendous display of culture, art, and beauty, and containing the largest collection of artworks I've ever seen. There were four museums gathered in one representing art from old masters of modern art at the end of the century, and surrealist art, with paintings by Rene Magritte.

We returned to Amsterdam extremely satisfied with our one-day tour in Brussels and planned the next itinerary. We decided to go back to Germany and visit Heidelberg, as well as return to Bern, the capital of Switzerland. I was thrilled to see Heidelberg as it is a well-known university town. When we arrived in Heidelberg, people in the street gave us directions to take a tram, and then walk down a pedestrian street. I always booked hotels close to the train station, so an hour of walking with backpacks seemed too long. Finally, we arrived at the Marriott Hotel, and asked at the reception about the location of the place in relation to the train station. We learned that we had been given the wrong direction. At least we knew how the pedestrian street looked like, lined with shops, and with the city's landmarks of Town Hall, and the Church of the Holy Spirit, where we stopped to say a prayer and catch our breath. Leaving the hotel, we discovered close by a picturesque river with old bridges. The Karl Theodor Bridge was an impressive 18th-century arch bridge, from where a path led to castle ruins on a hill. We ended the day at a local outdoor restaurant where we had schnitzel and German beer.

A couple of days later we were on a train to Bern, Switzerland. Bern is a city of fountains, one hundred of them, lined on Market street, and each one of them has colorful figures telling stories of different times. The most known Kronos Fountain of Greek mythology caught my eye. The figure looked fierce, as if devouring a child, which he did, according to the myths, to keep his children away from the throne. There was a statue of a bear standing in a fountain with a cub eating grapes close to the Clock Tower. The bear, wearing a helmet and with a banner and shield in his paws, was a symbol of the city.

I was happy to discover that the fountains had drinking water where you could quench your thirst on a hot summer day. Soon we reached a bridge over the Aare River, and looking down, I was stunned at the beautiful sight. Its clean dark turquoise waters were flowing in a strong current, and there were houses on its banks in a garden-like setting. What was peculiar was that there were people swimming down the river who held bags with their clothes over their heads. When they reached their destination, they swam towards the riverbank and took stairs to get out of the river. We decided to have a small picnic and got a melon from a close by fruit market. As a goodbye, we were serenaded with Rama Indians chanting for hours in the evening by the hotel.

France was next on our list. We had a quick coffee in the morning and hopped on the train for Lyon. As we were looking at the map, a lady walked over and asked us if we needed help. Contrary to the common belief that the French are not friendly, this woman was very polite and helpful. She bent over and pointed out on the map the locations of the places that we needed to visit. "You need to go first to the hill Fourviere, as it is there that the city originated in Roman times. Take a funicular and get off at the second stop at the Basilica. Our Basilica is like Montmartre in Paris. It overlooks the city and is its symbol. The Virgin Mary saved the city from a plague in the 1600s, and from invasion in the Franco-Prussian War. You should be here on December 8th, the day of the Immaculate Conception, when the whole city is lit up by candles thanking the Virgin."

Arriving in Lyon we headed to our hotel, which I booked the night before. I knew it was a short walk from the station, but we ended up walking in a circle for close to an hour. I wasn't going to tell Mitt, who assumed the role of a leader, to stop and look around as we passed the hotel a couple of times. We finally got ourselves situated. The hotel was clean and had all amenities, including air conditioning. And I could close the windows without hearing any of the noise from outside. Getting a map from the desk, we knew where to go, La Basilique Notre Dame de Fourviere and la Cathedrale Saint Jean Baptiste. The best part of the walk was reaching Old Town by crossing a bridge over the Saone River. As I was taking a picture of the magnificent Fourviere hill a young French couple kissed and waved at me, reminding me of how uninhibited and happy the French people are. We could hike but we opted to take the funicular. Stepping off it we saw the grandiose building of The Basilica, dominating Fourviere Hill and offering an incredible view of the city below. Mont Blanc, the highest peak in Europe, could also be seen in the distance. We also managed to walk by the Ancient Roman theatre, which unfortunately was closed.

Next stop was La Cathedrale, conveniently located at the bottom of the funicular in the Vieux town. At the end of a narrow street facing the square stood out the cathedral with its beautiful stained-glass windows, in an imposing Gothic-Romanesque style, dedicated to John the Baptiste. Once inside we discovered the famous, still working nine-meter-tall Lyon Astronomical Clock from the 14th century, with several dials, of which I remember the sun and the moon, and a calendar in the front. From there we headed to a restaurant in Vieux Quarter. Here I indulged myself in savoring *magret du canard*. I love duck dishes, and this one was delicious with duck breasts in sauce and with rice and vegetables in the middle. Mitt had *thon mi-cuit*—lightly cooked tuna with sesame in special sauce, and of course, we finished the meal with crème brulee, my favorite dessert. We returned to the hotel in the evening, happy and excited from the memories we collected during the day, and of course, we talked about places to visit on the next day. Lyon is in the Rhone Valley wine region, and I wanted badly to go to a winery, more specifically, in the Beaujolais region. Nouveau Beaujolais is the wine I always follow when it becomes available in the States in the fall. I prefer its taste from my younger years because it is light and dry, leaving a refreshing taste in the mouth. Unfortunately, it was not possible to visit this winery at short notice, so we decided to visit the medieval city of Perouges, which was built in the 1100s.

Early on the next morning, after fresh croissants and café au lait, we headed to the train station, and soon we were on our way. It was a short trip, about half an hour long. We got off the train at a small and cute French provincial train station and followed the signs for the city, which was perched on a hill with medieval walls around it. We walked on dirt roads by small country houses and climbed a hill to reach this amazing ancient place, which was surrounded by huge fortress walls. I had my eyes wide open when we entered through the lower of the two medieval gates. It was like walking back in time on cobblestone narrow streets, lined with houses of medieval architecture. The path led to a square with a church, an old inn, stores, and restaurants around it. The majestic linden tree, I learned from the waiter of a restaurant, was planted during the French revolution, which gave the name of the square—La Place du Til-leul. I noticed that door entrances were low, explaining the fact that people of medieval times were quite short. I was also curious why the old windows and doors were sealed. "The story behind it," explained the waiter, "is that once the spirits left, they were not to go back in." Here, at this unique restaurant of medieval structure, I had the best salad bar I've ever had, with delicious hot and cold hors d'oeuvres dishes paired with a glass of Beaujolais wine.

After lunch we continued our walk and reached the second gate. We wandered through the village, admiring, and absorbing every detail of the atmosphere around us. "Look at this bakery," I pointed out as a girl was selling the popular Perouges galette, which we had to try. At the end of the day, exhilarated from the unusual and beautiful experience at this charming and historic place, we headed back to the train station.

Returning to Lyon we stopped at the railroad station and booked tickets to travel on the next day to La Spezia, Italy, from where we planned to visit the Cinque Terre villages. My husband, who assumed the role of arranging reservations for the trains, approached the counter and requested information in English, to which the young lady responded in French that she did not speak English. He asked for her manager, and she responded that the manager did not know English, either. Wasn't he lucky that I spoke French? Besides, I love practicing the language.

We arrived in La Spezia and used GPS for directions. We started to walk from the train station towards the hotel, but to our surprise there was an apartment building at this address. The entrance had big wooden doors, and there was no sign with the name of the hotel that I booked the previous evening. We did not see a bell, and while wondering what to do, the door opened and an elderly woman appeared, with a basket in her hands. She explained that the fifth floor was rented to tourists, so we snuck in and looked around. There was a beautiful white statue of a woman in the middle of an enclosed yard. The elevator was very small, which was alright, since we had only backpacks. We got off on the fifth floor, and here we saw the name of the hotel. We rang the bell, and a young Asian girl opened the door. She was very pleasant and let us into a foyer from where we called the manager. While waiting for him, the girl explained that she was staying in one of the rooms and that she was on vacation. The manager arrived shortly and apologized. He showed us to our room, which was clean and comfortable with all necessary facilities, and that was all that we cared about. Later in the evening we strolled down the pier and had a seafood pasta, which one can have only on the coast of Italy. This time the meal was paired with Pinot Grigio. We returned to the hotel, excited to plan our visit to the five remarkable, world-renowned villages of Cinque Terre.

We rose early in the morning, eager to start our adventure. It was already crowded at the train station, but it was a short ride. We decided to start at the most remote village, Monterosso, dating from the ninth century. Getting off the train we immediately spotted the Aurora Tower. Further down was a marvelous medieval castle with elongated walls and round towers, and the 14th century St. Baptiste Church. The beach was extremely attractive and inviting, with umbrellas and lounge chairs to keep you out of the sun. But we decided to continue and hike to the next village, Vernazza. We climbed up a steep path by the sea, watching the Monterrosso village and beach disappear in the distance. The trail was breathtaking, with a view of the crystal blue sea water to the right and Mediterranean flora such as samphire, shrubs of thyme, rosemary, and lavender as well as chestnut and pine trees on the left. The hike was moderately strenuous, with the path becoming steeper in some parts. I was so exhilarated by the beautiful scenery, breathing in the fresh sea air, and smelling the aroma of the wildflowers. There was a booth on the way to Vernazza, where we paid a fee to enter the village, which we thought was the prettiest of the five villages. We saw it from the top of a hill, with colorful terraced houses, snuggled between rocky cliffs, that enclosed a part of the sea. We were all sweaty and hot, and we hurried down to go for a swim. There was no beach, but we found a secluded place to change and plunged into the cool Mediterranean Sea. We immediately felt refreshed, and still in wet bathing suits, headed up a steep narrow street. We reached a square, where we were attracted by the smell of freshly cooked fish at one of the restaurants.

After lunch we took the train to the third village, Corniglia, which had its own unique setup. Getting off the train we had to climb a few hundred steps to the village. Corniglia offered us another beautiful sight of an ancient Gothic church from the 12th century, and old colorful houses around it. There was a magnificent view of the entire region from the sea to the rolling green hills with Mediterranean vegetation. Hopping on a train we reached the fourth village, Manarola. We got off the train eager to see how it looked like and what it had to offer. A steep cobblestone street lined with colorful houses took us to the top, which revealed a breathtaking view of cliffs by the sea, and a small harbor with fishing boats. It was close to dinner time, and we stopped at a stand selling fried fresh fish. I knew from the Black Sea that such a meal is very delicious. Dinner was superb, and we cheered to the beautiful day with white Italian wine. We returned to La Spezia full of emotions and remarkable memories of the picturesque Cinque Terre villages. The second day we visited by train Riomaggiore, the fifth Cinque Terre village, and we returned to Monterosso for a day on the beach. All villages shared a panorama of colorful, attractive houses, but the layout for each one was different. Riomaggiore had a V-shaped indentation of a rocky hill, and a cliff over the water. We spent the rest of the day at Monterosso Beach, relaxing after the intense and fast-paced sightseeing of the previous day.

Later, in the afternoon, we stopped at the railway station to book reservations for our next destination, Arezzo in Tuscany. We picked this city which was not on any tourist pamphlets because it was halfway to the Amalfi Coast. We left early in the morning, feeling refreshed and in great spirits. I have loved ever since my childhood train rides, because that is a very pleasant way to get to know the countryside. And this trip was extra special, because we were going to Tuscany, the wine-producing region of Italy, with rolling hills of never-ending vineyards. Arezzo surprised us with its ancient history and architecture. The city was built in the ninth century, and had its charm from the past, but it also had contemporary shops. Our hotel was an old, attractive house on the main street. We were eager to explore the town, so we dropped the backpacks in our room and headed out on cobblestone streets, which took us to a square. From there we hiked to the top of a hill and were astounded by a magnificent view of vineyard estates. The Arezzo Cathedral dominated the hill with the nearby Basilica di San Francesco. We ended the evening with a perfect pasta meal and a glass of Pinot Grigio, the wine of the region. This city was a rival to Florence without the tourists, which we welcomed after the crowds in Cinque Terre.

In the morning we enjoyed a cup of delicious cappuccino with a croissant, and with backpacks on our backs, headed to the train station to reach the next city on our itinerary, Salerno. The hotel I chose was bed and breakfast on Corso Vittorio Emanuele. We walked all over the city and to the harbor until dusk, when we came across a very intimate restaurant. Here we finished the day with delicious pasta and vino Toto. The second day we took a boat to Positano, a city built on cliffs alongside the coast with views comparable to those in fairy tales. We walked up stairs on cobblestone streets and admired the ancient colorful homes with flowers. Earlier in the day we bought delicious cheese with pistachios, Italian salami, and freshly baked bread, and we had a delicious picnic on top of the hill. And I could not resist going for a swim before getting on the boat to Amalfi. That night we were happy to find a restaurant offering meals with fresh fish, like the one we had at Cinque Terre. We were strolling back to the hotel when we met an elderly couple from Arizona. They shared that they were on the Eurail for three months, which I thought was amazing as I believed that our one-month train trip at our age was extraordinary. The third day we took a train to Napoli, from where we transferred to Pompeii, a city of the world's worst tragedies. The place was buried in ashes from the eruption of Mt. Vesuvius in 79 AD and was restored over fifteen hundred years later to its present look. There were ruins of Roman villas with beautiful frescoes, a brothel, and upscale residences, roman temples, Roman bath houses, and an amphitheater. I was impressed with the statue of centaur, half human, half horse from Greek mythology. They also preserved burned bodies. I heard a story from a tour guide that an archaeologist in the 1800s discovered soft ashes, and by pouring plaster in soft cavities in the ashes, the bodies were restored, providing a very authentic picture of what occurred. "There were survivors in Pompeii," we overheard a guide say, "but the gladiators were not let out, because even in this tragedy, the ruling class was afraid that they would escape and cause problems."

The island of Capri was also on our list of places to visit. On the next morning we took a boat to the island, and soon it appeared in the distance with a striking beauty. It seemed that the island had a lower and upper part with houses, restaurants, and shops. A funicular took us to the top, from where the view was stupendous. My eyes wandered from the square below to the beautiful blue waters as I wanted to remember this amazing city forever.

We walked on the upper level of the island on narrow cobblestone streets; we climbed winding stairs and admired houses of old and modern unique architecture. We had a picnic, and then stopped for Italian cappuccino, which was so delicious that I still remember it. There was no time for more exploration, so we took the boat back, and stopped at Amalfi, a place just as picturesque as Positano. We walked by the harbor and stopped at a restaurant across from a ninth-century cathedral. We traveled at a fast pace, and I had so many wonderful places to remember. I closed my eyes, trying to memorize the sight of Amalfi. We ended the day in Salerno with wine and fruits from a market close to the hotel.

Our Italian adventure ended with a train trip to Bari from where we planned to take an overnight ferry to Greece. During our travel I realized that the trains in Italy are always late, but you still arrive at your destination. We had lunch at the port of Bari and headed to the ferry. I noticed that it had seven floors. We took a cabin for two; it did not have windows but was quite comfortable. At dawn we had coffee and yogurt and prepared for disembarking. I had reserved a hotel in the outskirts of Patras the night before, and we took a taxi to the resort. We walked straight to the beach and admired the early morning sunrise of spectacular colors over the water. The only disadvantage was that there was no sand, but the comfort and the delicious food at the hotel made up for it. We started to plan the upcoming trip and decided to find out how to reach Athens.

On the next day we took a small train to Patras for a fifteen-minute ride, and discovered that there was a Kiato bus going to the railroad station for Athens. We returned to the hotel happy that we figured out how to continue our trip. We studied the map and decided to break up the trip to Thessaloniki and stop at a beach resort, Katerini. The morning Greek-style breakfast was delicious. We were already packed and ready for our next adventure. We were no longer in Western Europe. For some reason we could not get first-class seats on the train to Athens and stayed in the dining car. A lady with a dog invited us to her compartment and we made friends, taking photos and explaining our trip to her. Katerini was crowded. There were tourists returning from the beach, walking down the main street in bathing suits, and kids dragging their beach toys. Our hotel was on the water, and the owner, who was Russian, told us that the rooms were clean, but not luxurious. This was not a concern as all we needed was a comfortable room. In the evening we had a very tasty dinner of fresh sea fish, Greek salad, and an ouzo drink at the next-door restaurant. The beach was overcrowded in the morning, but we managed to get an umbrella and chairs and enjoyed ourselves watching people happily running in the water, laughing, and having fun. A Bulgarian couple was sitting close to us with whom we made friends and exchanged addresses to stay in touch. The woman and I took a walk on the beach and talked about our lives. It felt like we had known each other for a long time. We stay in touch on Facebook, and we hope to meet again one day. That night was the last night of our trip, and we had another splendid dinner. But we did not stay up late because there was a long train trip to Sofia ahead of us on the train to Athens via Thessaloniki. This train was like a tram with a lot of stops. We finally arrived in Thessaloniki and started to look for a train to Sofia. I am not sure that paying extra for a sleeping car was worth it, because there was a nauseating smell in the compartment caused by the fumes. Even the open window did not help, but luckily, this trip was only for one night. Early in the morning the train pulled into the Sofia train station where I was happy to inhale the familiar smells of morning baked banitsas and coffee.

In summary I can say that this trip was an adventure that offered amazing sceneries and experiences from the mountain tops of the Swiss Alps to the Amalfi Coast. We explored cities of diverse histories and cultures from Belgrade to Amsterdam and back to Greece. We saw museums with spectacular artwork of world-famous artists, for which I provide information in another chapter. It was a fun trip, but I need to stress that we had to be very organized. We planned daily our itinerary and made reservations for trains and hotels. This was a budget trip as I used booking.com, expedia.com or hotel.com, looking for decent and not luxurious hotels. We also had a lot of picnics with freshly baked bread, fruits, and cheeses. In addition, I did not mind carrying only a backpack, as I felt like a teenager, and besides, it was very convenient because of all the train rides and extensive walking. European Eurail is an experience that I recommend to all young people and those young at heart.

CRUISING SCANDINAVIA

July is one of the hottest months in San Antonio, Texas, so I more than gladly agreed to join Mitt on an Oceania cruise in the Scandinavian countries. The cruise started in Oslo, Norway. We decided to arrive a few days earlier to get acquainted with the city, its surroundings, and the famous fjords. The first day we took a ferry from city hall to the Kon Tiki Museum, famous for the display of the wooden raft called Kon-Tiki, built in Peru, and used to cross the ocean, and the papyrus reed boats Ra and Tigris. Across from Kon-Tiki, on the same peninsula Bygdoy, was the Fram Museum. The museum was famous because of its large wooden, polar ship, described to be the strongest, and used in the Arctic and Antarctic regions in the late 1800s by Norwegian explorers. Both museums are a dream come true for an adventurer, who can visualize the crews on rough waters, meeting their challenges and conquering the seas. The ferry ride back to the city was very pleasant with picturesque scenery, which, as we approached the shore, was replaced by the outline of the City Hall with its two towers.

We arrived in the city on time to do some more sightseeing. First we headed to one of the world's most important buildings for commemorating peace, the Nobel Peace Centre. We were both very curious and interested to see it. The interior contained exhibits of every year's prize winners. The ceiling was attractive with paintings of people at work. I love palaces, so we walked to the Royal Palace, a magnificent building with columns in the front, offering a view of the entire city. It was a thrilling experience to visit the Oslo cathedral, dating from the 1600s, with celling paintings by Mohr and stained glass by Vigeland. We walked by the old church walls and came across galleries, souvenir stands, and cafes, which took us back to our contemporary lives. Then we strolled down a street towards the Oslo opera house. It was a magnificent modern structure. I was stunned by the Italian marble, and the white granite angled exterior. The pavement, which extended to the sea, had a line, separating Oslo from the water, or from the entire world. We walked around the building and on its roof, which was the main attraction that provided a spectacular view of the city from different angles.

The Akershus Medieval Castle and Fortress were the last stops on our list. We headed on foot to this place full of history, expecting a marvelous experience. The castle was a private residence for the king in the 1600s, but it was also a prison. Currently, part of the castle houses the Ministry of Defense and has an office for the Prime Minister. There were also museums of the resistance, and the armed forces, where tourists could receive a history lesson. I particularly enjoyed the grounds, which offered a beautiful view of the harbor and the city.

We returned to the hotel exhausted but energized by the sights we saw and the memories we collected from this city of the Vikings.

We were happy that we managed to do a full tour of the city's most remarkable places in one day. Now we were ready for a trip to the most world-renowned Norwegian fjords. We researched on the internet how to get to the Geiranger Fjord by public transportation and decided to take a train, which would allow us to see the countryside. The scenery was extremely picturesque. At one spot we arrived at a place with a huge waterfall, fiercely gushing down the Trollstigen Mountain, amidst green shrubs, wildflowers, and trees. The train stopped and the conductor asked all passengers to get off. We were pleasantly surprised when we stepped on the platform and heard beautiful music. We looked up towards the waterfall and saw a beautiful woman in a white dress, graciously dancing. Her body was like a vision appearing and disappearing in the white foaming waters of the falls. After this amazing sight we reached the town of Andalsnes, from where we caught a bus for Geiranger. That was the place where we boarded a boat to view and admire one of the nature wonders of the world. The boat was packed, but I managed to squeeze in the front of the deck, to better enjoy the changing scenes. There was a mist in the air, and a fog had enveloped part of the mountain, but nonetheless the sight was breathtaking, with the water weaving its way in between steep rugged land on both sides. Our return was adventurous because there were no assigned seats for the bus or a place where the people would line up for it. This was the last bus for the day, and we absolutely had to get on it, to be able to embark on our cruise ship on the next day. Mitt is a big man, and we had no problem with catching the bus, and even finding seats on it. I hadn't noticed when we arrived in the morning how narrow and steep the road was. My eyes were wide open on the way back as the view was amazing, but I was a little concerned because the bus was descending at a relatively high-speed close to the edge of the road. We took back the same picturesque train and arrived in the city excited by our impressions of the incredible fjords.

We felt very comfortable when we got on board the cruise ship in the morning. We had used Oceania cruise line a few times before and were familiar with their ships and programs. Stockholm was our first port of entry. The ship anchored further from the center, so we took a bus from the harbor to the city. Others went to explore the islands, but we wanted to see the Swedish capital. Stockholm has a fascinating history. It originated in the 13th century as a fortress by a point where Lake Malaren meets the Baltic Sea. Over the years the city spread out dramatically over dozens of islands and currently has five distinct districts. Stockholm is the capital of Nobel Prize awards, and the city hall was the first place we headed to. The City Hall building serves as municipality, and is also famous for its ceremonial halls, particularly the Blue Hall where the Nobel Prize banquet is held. The Blue Hall is not blue at all, as its walls are bare bricks, and the Golden Hall's name is derived from the gold mosaics surrounding it. I was impressed with the painting of Lake Malaren's Queen, holding a model of Stockholm in her lap.

The building had a majestic appearance, with a tall tower in between two sets of lower-level buildings. It is surrounded by islands and the shores of Lake Malaren, which provide a magnificent view. From there we ventured to the grounds of the royal palace, also situated by the water, which we viewed just on the outside, considering the little time we had. I was happy to take my photo with one of the guards. Then we continued down the narrow cobblestone streets of Old Stockholm, with houses dating from the 16th and 17th centuries and baroque doorways with rusting coats of arms. We followed a map with all worthwhile sightseeing places and walked by the Coronation church, with an extravagant exterior, to reach the Great Square. Here I noticed the stock exchange building with an unusual well in front of it. This was the end of a quick glimpse of the city in a period of a few hours. Stockholm deserves to be visited for a longer period, and we thought that we needed to return one day to get a better feeling of the city and to tour all the beautiful islands.

We traveled at night and arrived in the morning in different countries and cities. I woke up early the next morning and ran to the deck. We had arrived in Helsinki. There was an open market in the square by the harbor. I love walking in markets, and we made our way to it. There were stands with Finnish food, flowers, and souvenirs. People were sitting on benches having lively conversations. The brick Uspenski Cathedral at the square was an impressive building overlooking the harbor with its towers topped by gold cupolas. We headed first to the most recommended sight, the Helsinki Lutheran Cathedral. It was a very beautiful, imposing structure in the middle of the city at Senate square. We could spot it from a distance with its tall green dome, four smaller domes, and big white columns in front. It reminded me a little of Montmartre, as we sat on the stairs outside it. There was a wedding, and the cathedral was not open to the public. A monument of the Russian Emperor Alexander (1818–1881) was in the front, commemorating Finland's independence from Russia, which was initiated by the Russian king. It wasn't a big city, and it was easy to get around. We visited the Rock Church, its name derived from the fact that it was built into a rock. Here we managed to peek into its circular interior, sunbathed by the light coming from its dome. We approached downtown Helsinki and came upon a beautiful park, called Esplanada, that was lined with trees, fountains, and flowers. Here I was happy to see works of art, and the statue of the Finnish poet, Runeberg. We also ran over to Sibelius Park to see the recommended stainless steel-tube monument of the great Finish composer Sibelius. The stadium where the Olympic games were held in 1952 was close by, and we saw it as well. It was a day full of emotions. We saw outstanding buildings, parks, and the market, but most of all I appreciated this visit because President Ford signed an agreement in Helsinki in 1976 for uniting separated families from Eastern Europe and America, and Mom was allowed to come by me in the States.

Next on our itinerary was St. Petersburg, a city with palaces resembling those from fairy tales: The Hermitage, Catherina Palace, the Yusupov Palace, Peterhof Palace, and cathedrals renowned for their splendid beauty, and interior boasting in art history. We could not venture on our own without visas, so we booked tours for the couple of days while we were docked on the Neva River. It was a tough decision, but we picked to visit the St. Petersburg Cathedrals, the Peterhof Palace, as well as spend an evening at the ballet. While we toured the cathedrals we could take a glimpse of this city, full of history, and amazing architecture. We arrived at the St. Isaac Square in the center of the city and saw Nicolas the First's monument and the legislative Assembly. There was the magnificent Isaac Cathedral, named after St. Isaac whose saint day, May 30, coincides with Peter the Great's birthday. The exterior was decorated in a typical Russian style with gray and pink stone. The large central dome was covered with gold, and there were other smaller domes. Its interior was just as stunning. A sculpted white dove was suspended under the dome, representing the Holy Spirit, and the church boasted impressive 19th century art. The icons with stones of different colors were skillfully placed in the paintings. The iconostasis was of white marble with three rows of icons that surrounded the royal gate. Multicolor marble was used for the floors, and the semi-precious stones added to the sumptuous look of the cathedral.

The bus continued down busy streets, and we arrived at the Kazan cathedral, another building with a splendid display of beautiful columns, and a dome. The tour guide told us an interesting story. After Napoleon was defeated, the place became a pantheon of Russian glory, as keys of cities taken by the Russian army were still in there. The interior was dazzling like the Isaac Cathedral. It had red granite columns and multicolored mosaic floors as well as works of famous Russian artists.

The Church of the Savior on Spilled Blood was another architectural marvel. It had a stunning exterior of cupolas, decorated with enamel. The multicolored decorations inside and outside of the church were very impressive. The church was built by Alexander III on the spot where his father was killed by terrorists.

The Saints Peter and Paul Cathedral was located inside a fortress. This is the highest Orthodox church, with an impressive sight of attractive architecture and noticeable by its huge bell tower. It was built under the reign of Peter the Great and is a resting place of Russian emperors, including the entire Romanoff family, killed by the Bolsheviks during the Soviet revolution in 1917.

During the communist regime, the St. Petersburg cathedrals were closed since religion was forbidden. This story is the same as the one I knew from my childhood in communist Bulgaria. I remembered how my mother used to sneak me into a church in Sofia to say a prayer and light candles.

The visit to Peter Hof Castle was spectacular. The bus drove by forests in the outskirts of St Petersburg and arrived at the majestic castle that overlooked the Marine Canal, which was used in the past by tsars to sail to Finland. A gold-gilded staircase was at the entrance, leading to a lavish room, decorated with royal portraits. There was an astounding exhibit of Russian porcelain. We saw the royal bedroom chamber visited by Catherine the Great, and an oak study used by Peter. The inside of the palace boasted luxurious furniture, paintings, and chandeliers. The guide said that the palace was destroyed during the Second World War by the Nazis and completely restored by volunteers who loved to preserve Russian history. There was a spectacular view from the terrace in the back of the palace, which reminded me of Versailles, because of its romantic alleys alongside landscaped gardens, ponds, and cascading fountains. I was very happy because we were on time to observe the musical show of the fountains.

I must admit that I did not expect such splendor. I left very impressed with Peter Hof palace, a grandiose monument of Russian history.

I was looking so much forward to the Russian ballet in the evening. I could not see it in Moscow during my work assignment for the International Monetary Fund, as the ballerinas were on strike, and instead I saw an opera at the Bolshoi theatre. But here we were to witness one of the most cherished performances of Russian culture dating from centuries ago. We saw the famous *Swan Lake* and were astounded by the marvelous performance. I had seen *Swan Lake* as a student in Belgrade, but the Russian ballet performance is superb and breathtaking. A young girl served champagne during the intermission and was so happy to hear Mitt and I speaking Russian.

This week was a Russian navy holiday, and we saw Russian navy ships and submarines on the Neva River. It appeared that they were getting ready for a celebration, and we took photos. We could not venture on our own, but we still experienced the best of Russian history and culture visiting cathedrals, churches, Peter Hof Palace, and attending a ballet.

We woke up on the next morning, and from the terrace of our cabin I recognized in the distance Tallinn, Estonia, with its buildings with steeples. We did not book any tours, and we started our walk from the harbor towards the Old Town. We passed modern as well as attractive 19th-century narrow houses with pointed roofs in a triangular shape. Following the route, we approached the medieval city walls and walked through the Nun Gate with a high rising tower next to it. It was quite of an experience to go back in time to the Middle Ages as we entered the medieval city. We walked down cobblestone streets lined with amazing medieval houses and expected to see people coming out dressed accordingly with attire suitable for those times. I was very excited when we walked up to the picturesque St. Catherine passage and saw the inner yard with the Dominican stone monastery and the St. Catherine church dating from the thirteenth century. We looked around and noticed a wall from where we admired the best views of the city with its charming houses. I couldn't help noticing a statue of a praying nun, close to a wall with a writing, "breathe baby."

We couldn't resist and peeked in St. Nicolas and St. Olaf Churches, a short walk from there. Churches provide me with tranquility, and calmness, and on all my trips I made sure I included them in our itinerary. They also play important roles and are a part of history.

114

Mitt and I agreed that Tallinn is a charming historic city which we will remember.

We spent the next day in Gdansk, Poland, which is a Polish historic city. Its medieval gothic St. Mary church is the world's largest brick church. We walked through the Golden Gate, a decorated arch, which once was the entry to the city. From there we walked down a street lined up with spectacular buildings with elaborately decorated roofs. Neptune's Fountain was a reminder that the sea is close by. I wanted to have a souvenir from this place and bought a pair of amber earrings, which is the typical jewelry of the region.

Next on the tour list was Denmark. We docked at Copenhagen Harbor, which brought memories of my work as a tax advisor in 1995. I taught a class for a week at the OECD training center on auditing value added tax to Eastern European government officials. We got off the ship and I joyfully ran down the dock to the street by the canal, which leads to downtown. Mitt and I passed the famous Mermaid monument, and hurried alongside colorful colonial homes, outdoor restaurants, bars, shops, impressive boats, and yachts in Nyhavn District. There were people sunbathing and jumping in the canal, which we heard had water clean enough to drink, due to the use of a special purifying system. We continued to the pedestrian section, and I looked around. I remembered a Sunday morning in the fall of 1995 when I strolled out of the hotel to get fresh air. I recognized the café where I had cappuccino while talking to a local family. It seemed so long ago. We visited a museum, which I described in another chapter, and then took a boat back to the ship. It was a splendid day and we sat on the deck enjoying the sun.

Skagen, an old fishing village in Denmark, was the last stop on the cruise. It was a weekend, and everything was closed, but the word got around that a cruise ship was in the harbor, and soon the streets were full of vendors with stands for food, drinks, souvenirs, and clothing. There was even a band in the square. Mitt and I rented bikes and peddled through town, as we passed painted houses mostly in yellow, towards the place where the North and Baltic Seas meet. There was a lighthouse that we spotted from a distance. I got off the bike and ran to the water. It was an incredible sight to watch the waves of the two seas meet by a long sandbar. It was a splendid sandy beach and a favorite vacation spot for the Danish. We peddled back, and Mitt decided to return to town. I didn't realize it until I came to a place where I had to cross over to the other side of the street. I did not have a watch on me and returned to town, where I found Mitt at the bike rental place.

We disembarked in England at Southampton and took a cab to downtown London. I felt a tremendous joy as I was finally in the city that I wanted to see when I was a teenager in Sofia and attending the English Language High School. I was in London in the early '90s with my daughter Vanesa, but we had time only for a tour on a double-decker bus, and now I had the opportunity to visit all the places I dreamt of seeing as a young girl. Our hotel was by Trafalgar Square, a place I only read about and saw in magazines. I ran to the corner to see the National Gallery building, before we even registered at the hotel. It was still early in the day, and after checking in, we rushed out. We took a boat trip down the Thames, and I remembered the names of the bridges that my English language teacher talked about. The London Bridge, which I heard about as a child, and I knew a song about it, "London bridge is falling down," did not seem so spectacular. Tower Bridge, on the other hand, was very impressive. It could be seen from a distance with the two neo-gothic towers and a covered walkway between them. The enormous grey stones made it look medieval and grandiose. I was in awe looking at the Tower of London with city walls, adjoined to Tower Bridge. I knew that the next day I was going to take this trip on foot to take a closer look at the so-called Bloody Tower, which housed prisoners, and even prominent people, who were executed there. Unfortunately, we arrived late, and the tower was closed for visitors by the time we got there, but I managed to take a couple of photos of the yeomen warders who guarded the tower. On the next day we visited the grounds of Buckingham Palace and watched the changing of the guards, which was a spectacle with a special performance of the cavalry. We continued our tour to Big Ben, with its giant clock, and the Houses of Parliament, which resembled a palace. We also visited the National Gallery and the British Museum, which I describe in a separate chapter for museums in Europe. Hyde Park, which is mentioned in books and movies, was another place that I enjoyed tremendously, as I sat in a chair by the lake and watched the swans. From there I literally ran to see all the places that were dear to my heart: the Piccadilly Circus with its video display and neon signs; Abbey Rd., which is famous for the Beatles zebra crossing; Baker St., synonymous of the detective Sherlock Holmes, where the fictitious character supposedly resided; and Carnaby St. with its welcome sign for visitors to shop and stop at one of the notorious London pubs. London pubs are very cozy places as tables are very close to one another, and people chat with strangers. We entered one and sat at a table with a young man who told us that he was from the provinces on a business trip. We learned about his family, and his opinion about England getting out of the European Union. I had to experience one last thing, and it was a shepherd pie, which is an authentic English dish, and it was truly delicious.

Visiting London fulfilled my dream from my teenage years to visit England. Dreams always come through if you set your mind on them.

ACROSS SPAIN BY TRAIN

Spain was the last country we visited in the summer of 2019. Our plan was to start our trip from Seville and travel by train to the Basque country by making stops at other cities on the way. We made all arrangements on the internet a few days before our trip and chose the most incredible sightseeing places that we wanted to visit.

We took a plane from Sofia to Madrid, and from the airport we headed straight to the train station. The train from Madrid to Seville was fast, and looking out the window, the scenery was quickly changing at a speed close to two hundred miles per hour. We were in Seville for a few hours on a prior trip to Portugal, and in that short time we knew that we had to return and spend more time in it.

Our hotel in Seville was close to the famous Cathedral de Santa Maria de la Sede, considered to be one of the biggest cathedrals in the world, with beautiful architecture in Gothic style. Its Giralda Tower, which was a former minaret, stood solemnly up in the air with splendid views of the city. It is worth mentioning that the Giralda Tower was preserved, whereas the mosque of the Muslim Moors was destroyed when Christians retook the city and replaced it with a cathedral. The lines to enter the cathedral were extremely long, twisting around the corner, suggesting that the wait would be for hours. So, we decided to return the next day. We strolled through narrow streets lined with houses of Castilian architecture and came across a place offering a flamenco show, which we booked to see on the following evening.

Next morning, we got up extra early to beat the crowd visiting the cathedral, but to our surprise the cathedral was closed for visitors because of service. Mitt and I decided that this was an opportunity to attend Mass and at the same time see the cathedral.

"We are here for the service," we told the guard at the door. It was enjoyable to join other parishioners and take part in the service for a while. I am always overcome with peace and tranquility when I sit in any Christian place of worship, and since Mom passed away, I can even feel her spirit and presence. However, we were on a tight schedule and soon we had to leave. Walking towards the exit we saw the incredible interior which was like a place of art. There were paintings from Murillo, the most remarkable being *The Immaculate Conception* on the ceiling. I spotted another known artist, Francisco de Goya, with a painting of *Christ on the Cross*; Alonso Vasquez's piety paintings were also visible, as well as many more, which we had little time to admire under the scrutinizing eyes of the guards. The Royal Chapel was worth seeing as several kings were buried there, but most noteworthy was the tomb of Christopher Columbus, which we immediately recognized by the four figures representing the kingdoms of Spain at the time. I managed to take a photo, after which we had to leave. By that time there was a huge line waiting to enter, and the carriages for sightseeing tours were lined up in front of the cathedral.

Our next stop was Alcazar, where the line was also big, but manageable. There were girls from England on a weekend trip to Seville, chatting joyously. Alcazar, as a Royal Palace, with upper floors still reserved for the royal family, was very distinguishable from other castles in Europe combining Romanesque, Gothic, and Renaissance styles, the latter incorporating some Islamic elements of decorating. It's worth mentioning that it was built in the spot of a former Muslim Alcazar, which was destroyed after the conquest of Seville by Christianity. The Patio de las Doncellas with Islam inscriptions referring to Peter as sultan was a memory of those times. The long rectangular pool with reflecting images of the building and the sunken gardens by it, and reception halls alongside it, immediately grabbed my attention. It was a very beautiful sight, which I needed to capture in my photos. Salon de Embajadores, an ancient throne room, with tiled walls, was very much worth seeing. Its ceiling had a decoration resembling the sun, with spandrels filled with plant images. We carried a piece of this place in our hearts and took a lot of photos of the building and the gardens of immaculate design, with palm trees and fragrant flowers.

Plaza de España does not resemble any other plaza in the world. At the edge of a canal, it was surrounded by a palace curving around it, which was used for the city's administrative offices. In front of the buildings were fifty-two benches of frescos and colorful mosaics depicting the fifty-two Spanish regions.

Our visit to Seville ended with a flamenco show, where we noticed that at certain times the men would shout out the word *agua*. There is a drink, agua, in Seville, so I assumed it originated from there. A woman, in her forties, was moving graciously her body, and a man was following her closely.

Next morning, we hopped on a train to Granada, where we could see the only palace and fortress in the world of exceptional Islamic architecture, Alhambra. Our hotel was of a typical Spanish style in the downtown area and was at a walking distance to all sightseeing attractions. We were excited to be present at such a marvelous place, and as soon as we unpacked, we headed out and started to walk up a cobblestone street by a canal leading to Alahambra. We passed by charming old, well-maintained houses, with gardens in the front and beautiful flowers and bushes in bloom peeking from behind tall walls. It was getting late, so we resumed our exploration the next morning. Alahambra appeared in the distance as one building with a tower on the side. We were surprised when we walked in to see a complex of buildings with courtyards and fountains, the most beautiful was the one of the Lions. Alleys lined with trees provided the necessary shade on the warm summer day, and streams of water cooled the air, which was perfect for a pleasant walk.

Later we climbed on a hill by church St. Nicolas (Nicolas Mirador), which was across from Alahambra, to get the most beautiful view of this sight. After sunset we headed down narrow cobblestone streets to reach Caldereria, a place with shops, souvenirs, and tea stands. We continued our walk and reached a splendid cathedral, with the close-by Royal Chapel.

Our trip by fast trains took us next to the town of Zaragoza. Hotel Royal was luxurious and had excellent service. Our room was not ready when we arrived, and the receptionist offered us a complimentary dinner at the hotel's restaurant. The place was lively with a wedding reception going on, but they accommodated us, and I remember having the most delicious tapas, accompanied by Spanish red wine. The morning buffet was incredible with all imaginable Spanish specialties. But we were there to see the city, and soon we were on our way to Plaza Pilar. It was a weekend, and it seemed like the entire city was there engaged in different sports activities geared for all ages. There was a tower at the far end of the plaza, and we climbed it to get an excellent view of the area. We had researched the internet and next on the list was a visit to the Basilica de Nuestra Senora del Pilar with many colorful cupolas. Our last stop was at the 11th-century Aljaferia Moorish fortress palace, a UNESCO site. It was a long walk, and we stopped for a drink at a café halfway to the palace. Mitt forgot his backpack, but the server kept it safe and gave it to him on our way back. The palace itself was of marvelous architecture, with paintings on the ceilings and crafty ornamented pillars and walls.

Our next stop was Bilbao, which I wanted to see because of the gigantic flower-covered dog sculpture in front of the modern Guggenheim Museum. We stayed at a university dormitory, offered to tourists in the summer. Our room had a bunk bed, and I took the upper one. There was a modest break-fast in the morning with coffee. The place was clean and homey and re-minded me of my student life in Belgrade. In the morning we went straight to the Guggenheim Museum, with the giant spider statue in front. I walked around and came across the tallest and biggest flower sculpture of a dog, which was as tall as the building behind it. The museum itself was futur-istic with an unusual shape. It had stripes of silvery metallic pieces that were intermingled or wrapped around. It is an extremely modern concept of a structure which is not simple to describe. From there we headed to the old part of town, with winding, narrow streets, where we encountered col-orful buildings with architecture from different centuries, shops, and res-taurants. Here we saw the Gothic-style Santiago Cathedral, dating from the 14th century. It was lunchtime and we stopped at a restaurant by Plaza Nueva. Energized by the tasty meal and a copa vino, we went on a boat ride and saw all the sights down the river: the Guggenheim Museum with the spider statue in front, the market, Town Hall, and the reshaping of the area with the warehouses. Later in the evening we took the funicular to the top hill Artxanda and had a final view of this amazing city.

And since we both love beaches, our next destination was San Sebas-tian, a city known for film festivals. It was a big surprise to find out that we were on time to experience life in the city during an ongoing film fes-tival. We could not see any of the movies or events for which planning and reservations had to be made in advance, but we did get to observe the live-liness and the feverish excitement of parties carried on in the streets. Our hotel was across from the famous Playa de la Concha, a beach in the perfect crescent shape of a bay with hills on both of its sides. The statue of Jesus was on top of the one, which is like the statue in Rio de Janeiro, and on the other hill you can take a funicular to see the best views of the sea town re-sort. We chose to climb up the hill with the statue of Jesus, but it was later in the evening, and there was no direct access to it. Nonetheless, the hike was very pleasant with a walk in the woods, and we enjoyed the view of the city at night.

We always wanted to experience hiking at least at one of the parts of the Santiago Trail, so in the morning we headed from San Sebastian to the fisherman's village San Pedro, which was fourteen kilometers away, with steep paths along the sea and breathtaking views. I agreed to go on this trip partly because I expected to eat fresh fish in the village. We finally arrived, and we took a boat to get across to the village. Once we were there, we walked on narrow cobblestone streets and looked for a place offering fish meals. To my surprise all the restaurants were serving only drinks. What cheered me up was a village concert in the square, where local people were singing and playing Basque music. We were lucky to find a bus going back, as I was not looking forward to the difficult hike back to San Sebastian.

I could not be close to a beach and not visit it, so the day before leaving I headed to it in an extremely good mood. I was amazed at the big waves and figured out that it was not a day for swimming but lying in the sun and watching the people was just as pleasant.

After San Sebastian we traveled back to Madrid, and without spending much time anywhere else, we flew back to the States.

BACK TO FRANCE BY AIR, TRAIN, AND BUS

I had been to France as a French teacher with a group of my students and their parents, and later as a US tax advisor when I visited Paris frequently for meetings with the Director of the US Treasury Tax Advisory Program. And both Mitt and I stopped in Lyon during our EURAIL trip.

I love Paris, and I jumped with joy when Mitt suggested that we start our summer vacation with a trip to Paris and Bordeaux. I always wanted to visit French vineyards and was thrilled that this trip would include a famous wine-producing region. My choice of hotels was always a place in the center of events and activities, and for Paris I booked a hotel close to the opera house. We arrived in Paris in the morning, so we had the entire day to enjoy the City of Lights. Our visit to the museums is described in a chapter for European museums, so here I will talk about our walks and sightseeing. There is something very special about the bridges over the Seine, and I was so happy to visit them again. I took a deep breath seeing Pont Alexander with its marvelous statutes and lamps in Arts Nouveaux style; Pont Neuf, the oldest bridge, although *neuf* means new; and Pont des Arts. This bridge was known for the locks with inscription of people's names that they attached to its sides and then threw the keys in the water. This experience was not available anymore. The locks were removed because of their weight on the bridge. There was another place that I needed to see again, and that was the charming hill Montmartre. We walked up to Sacre-Coeur-Basilica and sat on the steps in front of it, eating a French gyro and admiring the marvelous view of the city. I've never been to Moulin Rouge, and on our way back we reserved tickets for its show. The popular and energetic leg-kicking dance called cancan, which dated from the late 1800s, was still a performance to remember.

No matter how many times I had visited Paris before, I still had to go on a boat ride on the Seine. It was sunset, and the sun illuminated the famous Paris landmarks of Tour Eiffel, Arc de Triomphe, and Musee d'Orsay. It was a beautiful way to end the day.

We both loved to wander the streets, doing sightseeing, and stopping for a tasty bite. The Paris streetside outdoor restaurants and cafes are a cultural experience where Parisians spend hours watching the crowds and relaxing as the tables and chairs are lined to view the sidewalks. Here I had the most delicious French onion soup and crème brulee.

On our free day we took a train to see the Dune of Pilat, described as the tallest and biggest dune in Europe. I was stunned by its size as it was huge and extended to the horizon. There were people on it who looked smaller and smaller in the distance. We were determined to climb to the top and get to the other side where we could reach the ocean and have a swim. There were steps on the way up, and it did not seem extremely difficult to climb up the hill. The view from the top was marvelous, overlooking Arcachon

Bay. The beach was so welcoming and inviting after the strenuous climb that I jumped in the water as soon as we descended the dune on the other side. We spent a few hours soaking in the sun and enjoying the scenery. However, it was somewhat more difficult to return. There were no steps on this side of the dune, and on the way up we walked in other people's footprints. We had to rest a couple of times, but we still managed to be on time to catch the last bus to the train station for Paris.

On the next morning, we headed for Bordeaux. The train from Paris to Bordeaux was a high-speed train which took a little over two hours at about two hundred miles per hour to reach its destination. I do not remember much of the scenery from the train. I knew that there were cute cities, but time did not permit to stop at any of them. I wanted to experience Bordeaux, a region of the famous French wine, so we booked a tour for an entire day. We traveled by bus and saw marvelous chateaux buildings of new and old architecture surrounded by acres of perfectly manicured vineyards. I was surprised to find out that *chateau* was the name for a house at the vineyards and not a castle. We stopped at a couple of vineyards to learn their processes of making wine, and I found out that the Bordeaux wine was a mixture of Merlot and Cabernet Sauvignon. We had Bordeaux wine during lunch at one of the chateaux, which had a pleasant taste. In the evening we took a walk from the hotel to the old part of town. We crossed the medieval century city door and found ourselves in a very attractive area with cobblestone streets with stores and restaurants. We walked past the town's Grand Theatre with huge columns and statues of gods, and the Sainte-Croix Church with attractive engravings of figures on the outside. We walked in, and I crossed myself. Then I looked around and noticed an impressive interior with columns and an old organ.

We had selected from the map to see Place de la Bourse, which is famous for its architecture and design. I was amazed by its view. The Bourse Palace was an impressive building, along with the Hotel de Fermes, with sculptures of Minerve and Mercury, and Hotel de la Bourse. The square itself was a masterpiece of history, ordered by King Louis XV at the edge of the River Garonne, and famous for the Mirror of Water (*Miroir d'eau*). It was so relaxing after running all over town to dip our feet in water and sit at the edge of the square, watching the boats on the river.

On the next day we headed to Saint-Émilion, a medieval city with wineries, which was a short bus ride from Bordeaux. I felt happy and smiled when we approached the city with chateaux amongst beautifully cared for vineyards. The old French teacher in me became alive and I enjoyed every minute of this trip. We arrived soon, and my eyes wandered to get a full view of the place. There was a Romanesque church with pointed arches that dominated the area surrounded by one-story modest houses. The city was charming with its cobblestone streets and views of vineyards for as far as you could see. I was particularly impressed that we could walk into a winery and have wine tasting without any prior arrangements. The owner gave us a tour and showed us the different wines that he produced, which I preferred to a lesson of wine producing. We returned to Bordeaux with a bottle of his best wines, which we enjoyed in the evening.

France is a country where I will return many times as it has so much charm. Whenever I visited it, I discovered new sights and had unforgettable experiences. The flight to Sofia was short, and after settling in Mitt's apartment, we planned a trip to Greece.

TRAVEL TO GREECE BY CAR, BUS, AND BOAT

I grew up in Bulgaria, but I never visited this neighboring country until now. In my young years travel from Bulgaria to capitalist countries was not allowed. In those days I was intrigued by life in Greece, its culture and sights. We could buy records of Greek music, which I found to be melodious and lively. It was by listening to Greek music that I became curious and dreamt of traveling to this land of ancient history and culture.

Forty years later my wish was granted. Mitt and I rented a car to drive from Sofia to Athens. We traveled to the Greek border, passing by the Rila and Pirin Mountains. This is a very picturesque region of mountain ranges, with the River Struma running alongside the road. There was a restaurant on the way offering fresh rainbow trout, and we could not resist stopping for a quick lunch. We reached the border in the afternoon, and I was amazed how easy it was to cross it. Bulgaria is now a democratic country, a member of the European Union, and it was sufficient to show only identification cards to enter Greece.

We reached by sunset a place called Kumata by the Aegean Sea with a fortress on the hill. The gold and red sunrays were playing in the water, inviting us for a swim before it got dark. We checked into a hotel and headed to the beach for a refreshing swim after the all-day car trip. Then we had a spectacular evening sitting on the terrace by the sea, where we tasted delicious Greek dishes in the calmness of the night and the pleasant breeze which caressed my face and shoulders.

We got up early in the morning and were struck by the amazing sunrise. The sun had the most beautiful fiery red color, covering the sky and reflecting on the still waters. Shortly afterwards we were on the road to our first destination, the Meteora monasteries. The sight was breathtaking. The monasteries perched high in the sky on huge rocks appeared magical, invoking deep spiritual feelings. A tour guide explained that they were built during the Ottoman Empire to preserve Greek Orthodox religion, and that the building materials were hoisted up in huge boxes alongside the cliffs. We walked up a steep path and reached the Great Meteoron, which was the biggest monastery with three separate churches. Then we climbed 186 steps to reach the Varlaam Monastery. It was a great hiking exercise, and the view was splendid. All six monasteries offered marvelous sights of the Pindus Mountains in the distance, and a cute town at their foothills. By noon we felt an inspirational energy and decided to visit another spiritual sight, which was the historic and incredible Greek town Delphi. This place was the worship site for Apollo, the Greek god of light, music, and healing, and the mythical Oracle, who was visited by pilgrims for healing advice. The complex was tucked in the Parnassus Mountains and overlooked a thriving ravine with a small meadow and beautiful Greek peony flowers, among other supra-Mediterranean vegetation. It was a spectacular sight which took us back in history with its amphitheater, ruins of temples, and an old soccer field at the top of a hill. We drove to town, which was very attractive with its old, narrow streets and a mixture of old and new buildings with stores and hotels in the center. The place was charming, and I wished we had more time to spend the night, but for this trip, our destination was Athens. We had lunch at a restaurant overlooking Delphi Lake and enjoyed the splendid view of the mountain region. In an hour or so we were back on the road, and by late afternoon we entered Athens. We found a room at the Hilton Hotel, which was conveniently located close to the Acropolis. I was eager to visit this city of rich history and stories about ancient gods and goddesses. We got up early in the morning, and after a traditional Greek breakfast, walked over to the Acropolis. We climbed on top of a rocky platform, and memories came back from my history books. I remembered the story about this place being sacred and devoted to the goddess of war and the city protectress, Athena. The Parthenon, a temple of the virgin Athena, was in the center. A theatre called Odeon of Herodes Atticus was close by, and next to it was a ruin of a temple. We had only one day, and to get a better picture of the city we hopped on one of the two story sightseeing buses. We saw the temple of Zeus (the god of all gods), which was a gigantic structure with some columns that suggested the existence of a good-size building in the past. There was a park in the back, next to the Parliament, that looked inviting on a hot summer day. We managed to take a glimpse at the ruins of Roman Agora, an ancient marketplace that was the main meeting place in the past. At the end of the day, we took a stroll in the picturesque neighborhood Plaka, which had narrow pedestrian medieval streets and attractive cafes and restaurants. I left Athens full of emotions because of the walk back in ancient history, with monuments testifying to what life had been ages and centuries ago.

Below are my memories of more sights in Greece which we visited at other times.

Santorini Island was a stop when we were on a Royal Caribbean cruise. As we approached land, I could see at the bottom the black soil left from an erupted volcano years ago. Above it there were beautiful all-white houses and churches with blue domes. We took a cable car from the dock to get to the upper part of Santorini, where we discovered how charming the island is, with cobblestone streets and outdoor cafes, restaurants, and shops. Beautiful flowers decorated the houses and added to an atmosphere of harmony and beauty. Santorini's white cave houses were particularly attractive. They were dug into the volcanic rock alongside the cliffs and were the island's major attraction. We had a few hours to spare, and decided to walk down to the port. On the way we met tourists on donkeys. This was not an attraction for me, as I grew up on my grandmother's farm surrounded by farm animals. There was a restaurant at the bottom where I had to try authentic Greek kabob and spinach pie. I left Santorini impressed by its beauty and charm.

During the same trip we stopped at Olympia, where we opted to go to the best beach, Platamonos, instead of touring the ruins.

On another occasion we booked a bus tour from Sofia to a four-star resort in the Chalkidiki region, which consists of three peninsulas lined up as fingers—Kassandra, Sithonia, and Athos. The bus ride was all right, except for the complaints of the Bulgarian passengers who were afraid of catching a cold from a draft. This was something I remembered from my childhood, and it still existed. The temperature of the air conditioning was turned up, and the windows were closed. It was stuffy, and I opened my window, which caused a big commotion. Our hotel was in Sithonia, the peninsula known for its picturesque landscape of vineyards, forests, a lot of green areas, and mountains. The hotel had a nice beach, and the accommodation was great. We wanted to explore and visit the other two peninsulas, so we booked trips for each one of the days on our vacation. First, we visited Kassandra, which is known for its nice beaches. However, we discovered that in summertime, Kassandra was so overcrowded that you could not find a place to put down your towel, let alone find an umbrella and a lounge chair. The town of Kallithea was cute, with shops and restaurants on the street by the beach, but again the place was packed with vacationers. The tour continued to another beach, which was not as crowded. Here there was plenty of room to lie down on the sand and go for a swim. We returned to the hotel, and I thought of how wonderful the boat ride was in the Aegean Sea with its beautiful turquoise blue waters.

The most interesting and memorable boat trip was the one to Athos, a peninsula with monasteries, where females are not allowed to visit. The boat was gliding slowly alongside the peninsula so we could take photos or simply admire the views of the monasteries. We were at a comfortable distance, which allowed us to look at the buildings and the surrounding area of forests and nature. The Russian monastery was the most impressive, with its colorful buildings and chapels with domes. Other monasteries were of equal beauty, such as Saint Paul Monastery and Dionysiou Monastery. The latter was an attractive building with terraced terrain reaching the sea. The monastery was dedicated to Michael and Gabriel with their statues on pillars in the front and was very attractive. The boat ride ended at a village with shops selling religious souvenirs and icons, and since my religion is Eastern Orthodox, I bought a couple of icons. At the end of the trip, I reflected on the experience of this Greek vacation and thought how beautiful Greece is with its scenery of sea and mountains, and how precious it is to visit such a country of amazing ancient history and culture.

PORTUGAL BY AIR AND CAR

Portugal always fascinated me with its history of exploration and discovery of routes to India, China, and Japan, with names of great explorers as

Vasco da Gama, Christopher Columbus, and Ferdinand Magellan. I read in geography books about the country's cold and rocky northern beaches, mountain ranges in the interior, and the beautiful Algarve in the south with famous sea resorts and lush vegetation.

We were on vacation in Bulgaria when we made on the internet reservations for our trip to Lisbon. We usually pick to stop at different cities in Europe before returning to the States and this year we chose Lisbon.We flew into Lisbon from Sofia and picked up the rental car at the airport. We were both curious about this city, with its preserved history from the times of the Celtic tribes, the Romans, and the Moors. Our hotel was by Jerónimos monastery and Belém Tower, both important city landmarks. We checked in and left in a hurry, eager to get acquainted with the Portuguese capital. The monastery was an impressive building, but we decided to visit it later. We passed by the Belém Tower, which is a fortification from the Renaissance century and is known as a place of embarkation and disembarkation of Portuguese explorers in the 16th century. In front of the tower was a tram stop, and we hopped on a tram heading for the center. From the tram I immediately noticed the decorative colorful tiles on the buildings' exteriors, which I heard about and saw in travel brochures. We got off at the square, Praca do Comercio, which was recommended at the hotel. The plaza was amazing. It was built by the water with King Joseph's statue in the middle. Across were yellow-colored buildings with arcades, and balconies on the first floor. From Comercio Square we walked through a majestic gate to Rua Augusta Street. Suddenly we felt that we discovered the pulse of the city. A very lively scene opened in front of us, with a mosaic pavement, restaurants, and shops. There were tables in the middle of the street with people having their meals, chatting, and laughing. We were curious to see more and continued our walk. Soon we reached Rossio Square, with elegant sidewalk cafes. There was an impressive monument in the middle with Dom Pedro statue on top. The fountains on each side of the baroque-style square added to its beauty. The atmosphere was very lively, with people sitting at the sidewalk cafes in the company of friends or relatives. Their happiness was contagious, and we decided to stop for a drink. We stayed for a while, amused by the scene of people around us who were gesturing and talking loudly in expressing their emotions. Afterwards we followed the city map to the amazing Rua Cor de Rosa. The street resembled a picture from a fairy tale. It was lined with a beautiful pink tar carpet, and colorful, attractive buildings with balconies. Later we read that this place was considered dangerous in the past because it was full of prostitutes and gangsters. Close by was the Santa Justa lift, which connected the lower part of the city from the Baixa District to Bairro Alto, Upper District.

Early on the next day we continued to explore the city. We followed a city map and started our walk from Commercio to Municipal Square, where we saw an uncredible palace of neoclassical style, with beautiful sculptures, currently housing the City Hall. I was amazed by the 16th-century church, Conceicao Velha, which was beautifully decorated with flowers and angels.

We returned to Baixa District and decided to walk to Bairro Alto, where we planned to see the Church of Sao Roque. We were surprised by its plain exterior, because the interior was magnificent, with beautiful mosaics on the ceilings and gilded decorations. The significance of this church was that it was built in honor of Vasco da Gama for his maritime discoveries.

We left the church very much impressed with its décor and history. From there we headed to Sao Jorge Castle, which was situated on a hill. We walked up enchanting cobblestone streets, lined with centuries' old houses, bathed in the late summer sun. The castle was a grandiose fortified building, and we were astonished to find out that its original construction dates from the sixth century. The place appeared very peaceful when we approached the main gate decorated by King Henriquez statue and cannons. We walked by the ramparts and climbed the towers, from where we discovered a spectacular view of the pastel-colored old city buildings, an estuary, and a suspension bridge. The atmosphere was so serene that we sat on a bench to rest in the beautiful garden with ancient olive trees. On the way down we stopped at Igreja de Santiago. This church had a simple exterior, whereas the interior boasted of astounding beauty. The altarpiece was covered with gold, there were gilded decorations, and the walls were tile paneled. It was getting late, and we stopped at a unique, intimate restaurant located by steps going down a steep cobblestone street. I do not remember the name of the place but there was an image of a rooster at its entrance. I am mentioning this place because here we had extremely delicious octopus and other seafood.

On the way back to the hotel Mitt pointed out from the tram the Edgar Moniz Hospital, named after a psychiatrist who received a noble prize for introducing lobotomy surgery as treatment of psychiatric disorders. It was our last day in the city, and it was time to visit Jeronimos Monastery by the hotel. At the monastery we learned that it dates from the 1500s. The building looked like a palace, with sculptures portraying maritime events in attractive forms and shapes. The church Santa Maria had an entrance of ornate design and unusual structures on both sides extending to the roof. The monastery was a historic monument with Vasco da Gama's tomb and tombs of well-known poets, historians, and former presidents.

In the morning, we drove south to the coast, admiring the scenery of changing vegetation from uncultivated lands and cork oak to olive and fig trees. We reached Faro, a city close to our resort, and before checking in, we drove by the cathedral and the old town area with cobblestone streets, charming houses, restaurants, and cafes. The place looked very inviting, but we had to find our hotel before dark. Our resort was by Praia da Falesia, which was not easy to locate, and we had to stop a few times to ask for directions. The AP Adriana Beach, an all-inclusive resort, was right by the beach, with a pool and pine trees in the front. We checked in and immediately headed for the beach. There was an amazing view past the pine trees of rust-colored cliffs overlooking the beach. We discovered the beauty of the beach in the morning when the sunrays bounced off the rocks and made them shimmer. It looked like millions of diamonds were among the ochre-and-cinnamon-colored surface. We took a long walk on the beach and admired the view of the sea with waves joyfully splashing on the sand and the red cliffs bathed in the sun.

After a couple of very relaxing and enjoyable days, we headed east to

Spain towards the city of Cordoba.

The drive was delightful, with beautiful Mediterranean vegetation alongside the road. We did not even know when we entered Spain. We stopped in Seville for a couple of hours and parked close to the Giralda Tower. It was noon, and it appeared that the sightseeing buses were not available. We walked into the city across the Almohad Wall, which surrounded the Old City, and ventured on cobblestone streets, with outside bars and people who seemed happy, talking and laughing over a drink. It was a very lively city, and we decided that we needed to return.

In the evening we arrived in Cordoba. Our hotel was in the old part of town on a very narrow street, and it was impossible to drive to it. We were lucky as we found another hotel close to the entrance of the Old Town.

Early in the morning, we ventured into the city. I loved the narrow cobblestone streets with souvenir stores, restaurants with tapas, and cafes with aromatic deserts. Soon we reached the Great Mosque. The mosque was converted in a cathedral in the 1500s and was a gem of Islamic architecture. We crossed a patio with orange and palm trees and walked into a hall with numerous marble and jasper columns with amazing arches. Our next stop was Alcazar Castle, with walls from the Moorish era and an inquisition tower which was built later. The palace had gorgeous gardens with beautiful flowers and ornamented fountains and pools. From Alcazar we walked on the Roman arched bridge where we observed a couple recently married in the company of friends, a sight that brightens any day.

Our next stop was in Badajoz, a city at the border with Portugal. This place is not on any tourist maps but is surprisingly attractive. A long bridge connected the city with the old part of town, where we encountered nightlife with restaurants and historic charm. Despite the fatigue, we managed to stroll on the cobblestone streets and reach the cathedral, which had the appearance of a fortress.

We arrived in Lisbon on the next day and drove straight to the airport, where we returned the car rental and took a plane back to the States.

ISTANBUL – A CITY WHERE EUROPE MEETS ASIA

It was one summer morning in Mitt's apartment in Sofia when he looked at me and said: "I want to have Turkish coffee at the Bosphorus."

It was easy to book a flight and find a hotel near Hagia Sophia on the internet.

The flight from Sofia to Istanbul was short, and soon we were on the steps of our hotel. The porter greeted us and asked for our names. This assured me that the security at the hotel was good. We had a nice room, and there was a restaurant on the top of the building with an amazing view of the Bosphorus, Hagia Sophia, and the Blue Mosque. The Bosphorus was full of life with fishing boats, speed boats, and yachts. The city was so vibrant that I could hear the loud voices of men and women from below, and I could see further away on the left side of the Bosphorus people who were swimming. The scenery was incredible, with buildings clustered to each other for as far as one could see. There was the Galata Tower and more minarets of mosques. It was noon, and we ordered Turkish delicacies and a drink called raki. We didn't want to waste any time and headed outside. We were both in Istanbul before, but we still had to go inside Hagia Sophia. Hagia Sophia was a museum for a while and was recently converted to a mosque. I had to see again its beautiful architecture and splendid display of art. Once the principal church of the Byzantine Empire, it was converted to a mosque by the Ottoman Empire. The building was a museum for a while and again converted back to a mosque. What is peculiar is that one could see the images of the Virgin Mary's and Archangel Gabriel's icons coming through the paint, a reminder of its origin.

From there we headed to the Blue Mosque, another building of architectural wonder. The inside walls are decorated with Iznik tiles of predominantly blue color from the city of Iznik, and there are beautiful flower designs at the gallery level of the mosque. Walking in, we were stunned by a beautiful display from the light, which came through the beautiful stained-glass windows, reflecting off the decorative carpets. Back in the street we headed to Topkapi Palace, which was built in the 15th century, and where sultans of the Ottoman Empire lived for centuries. There was a beautiful garden in the front with flowers, green meadows, and benches along the alleys. The marble building added to the beauty of the place. We both had been inside the palace, so we decided to visit only its restaurant for a cold drink and coffee. We sat on the terrace, and I tried to remember the interior, as I was sipping on Turkish coffee. The Harem was in the front, which was a place where the sultans kept their concubines and children who were locked in the luxury of the palace and were not allowed to step foot outside it. The sultan's quarters were in a third courtyard, a place which was extremely private for the sultan and his family. The entire interior of the place was dazzling with objects and decorations of Islamic art. From the palace, we strolled down the beautiful Gulhane Park. It was getting late, and we hurried back to the hotel as we had booked an evening dinner cruise on the Bosphorus. The ship parted at sunset, and we could enjoy the spectacular sights of the city, with sunrays bouncing off the water. We saw the bustling spice market, the Bosphorus Bridge, where I remember having fresh fish dinner during a prior visit with my daughter, grandson, and my cousin and his wife. Further along was a beautiful mosque, the glamourous Dolmabahce Palace, a tower in the distance, the Hagia Sophia, and the Blue Mosque. It was an unforgettable evening under the stars of one of the most attractive cities in the world.

Mitt's wish came through on the second day when we sipped Turkish coffee on the terrace of the hotel. It was prayer time, and we listened to the chanting of the Islam prayers from Hagia Sophia and the Blue Mosque. Later in the day we decided to peek at the Basilica Cistern, an underground hall with massive lit columns lined up in rows for storing water supply for as far back as the Byzantine Empire. Then we walked to the famous Galata Bridge, which was well known for its fish restaurants. We observed fishermen throwing their fishing rods in the water and watched the crowds of people by the spice market. It was amusing to just sit and observe the colorful hustle and bustle at the bridge. On the way back to the hotel we stopped at a restaurant and had an exquisite seafood meal with fresh fish. We ended the day by having popcorn and sweet corn in the square by the Blue Mosque and Hagia Sophia, surrounded by crowds of people and children laughing and having fun.

CHAPTER 14
Mediterranean Cruises

ROYAL CARIBBEAN CRUISES

The Mediterranean cruise was as exceptional as I imagined it from photos and from reading history books and magazines. I was looking so much forward to seeing ancient Spanish and Italian monuments and buildings and viewing the beauty of the Tuscany valley, as well as life in cities like Rome, Valencia, and Florence. Flights from the States to Europe always arrive in the morning, so we were in Madrid at dawn. This was my first time in Madrid, and the taxi driver was nice enough to stop for a moment in front of the Royal Palace so I could admire the majestic building and snap a couple of photos for a souvenir. We took the train to Malaga, planning to spend there a couple of days before the cruise. That was my first experience on a high-speed train, and the ride in the first-class compartment was most enjoyable. At a speed of 310 km/hour, we reached Malaga in two and a half hours, during which time we were served some of the best Spanish appetizers and drinks. There was a film festival in the city, and on the way to the hotel we saw a crowd in front of a building with a red carpet waiting for a celebrity. Later, we found out that the people were waiting to see Antonio Banderas. I was eager to explore this famous city on the Costa del Sol, and we immediately set off on our own after checking into the hotel. We stopped first at the cathedral, which was a majestic building of Renaissance architecture. Here I learned that the cathedrals in Spain were previously mosques, which the Christians converted to cathedrals. I briefly sat inside and enjoyed the marvelous decorative details and artwork. Alcazaba Fortress, which was a historic monument and dated from Moorish times, offered spectacular and memorable views of the city.

Then we walked down ancient cobblestone streets and reached a plaza with a beautiful fountain. It was lunchtime, and we stopped at a restaurant to try the famous authentic Spanish paella. I recognized Picasso's birth house at the plaza by his statue in front of it and was extremely happy to visit it and view the paintings of this prominent artist. I was particularly interested in learning about his evolution in painting styles from realistic to abstract. Constitution Plaza was worth seeing, with its beautiful palm trees and tall buildings around it, famous for the printed on the ground copies of the first newspapers of Spanish democracy. We ended the day with another beautiful view of the city from the defense walls of Gibralfaro Castle. Malaga left me with precious memories of its rich history, culture, and beauty.

The excitement continued the next morning when we packed in a hurry, checked out of the hotel, and boarded the ship, which was a huge floating vessel with all possible amenities. We situated ourselves fast in our stateroom, which I loved because it had a balcony, then participated in a mandatory safety drill, and visited all floors to get familiarized with the ship's layout. There was an ice show in the evening that we decided to see.

After a night at sea the ship docked in Valencia, Spain, a city which I was eager to discover for a long time. It was Sunday, and all the stores were closed, including the famous Central Market, which was the biggest one in Europe with the most exquisite food stalls. Nonetheless, we came across probably the only open food store in the city and bought some of the famous Spanish prosciutto and cheese. Then we stopped for a cup of cappuccino at a café by the market and enjoyed looking at people dressed for church and happily chatting. Valencia's cathedral was in the vicinity, and we headed in its direction. The building was outstanding with its mixture of architectural styles—Gothic, Baroque, and Renaissance. We hoped to see a bullfight, and we headed towards the Plaza de Toros, which dated from the eleventh century. The place looked empty, and the ticket office was closed, but we still managed to see the arena and visualize how lively and incredible it must be during a real bull fight.

Corsica was the next port where we docked. I noticed that some Europeans left the ship, while others got on it, and realized that they use it to travel for short distances. We wanted to see the capital, Ajaccio, and headed to its center. It was early in the morning, and the open market was full of fresh fruits, vegetables, and homemade cheeses. The aroma of French-baked breakfast rolls, crepes, and pastries filled the air with a sweet and heavenly smell. I smiled as I remembered my days of teaching French and taking my students to French cafes. The city was awake, and souvenir and food stores were open. We followed the winding narrow streets to the Place de Gaulle with Napoleon's statue and Maison Bonaparte, the emperor's birthplace. We visited the Cathedrale d'Ajaccio where Napoleon was baptized, and that concluded our historic tour. Corsica also has beautiful beaches and the blue colored crystal waters of the Mediterranean Sea are so attractive that I knew that I needed to return one day.

I woke up the next morning with a big smile. We were scheduled to visit Florence, the capital of art, fashion, and pasta dishes. I was ready in no time as I was anxious to visit this ancient city with historic buildings of famous Renaissance architecture. We disembarked at Livorno and took a train to Florence. I was amazed at the scenery of beautiful valleys, with vineyards and cypress trees lined up in perfect order with attractive houses on the properties. Once in town, we walked slowly not to miss a thing. Soon we reached Piazza de la Signoria, which is a glamorous square of history and art. There were local people and tourists who were admiring its beauty with Palazzo Vecchio, which is a medieval fortress, the Neptune's fountain, the Loggia del Lanza building, and the spectacular statues of famous Italian artists. We climbed to Piazzale Michelangelo, from where there was a beautiful view of the city with the dome of the Cattedrale di Santa Maria, the city's distinguishable landmark. Florence could not be mistaken for any other city in the world because of Ponte Vecchio on Arno—a medieval built-of-stone bridge, and the rolling Tuscany hills in the distance. Ponte Vecchio is the oldest bridge in Florence and is unique because of the artisan, souvenir, and jewelry shops on it, which are an attraction for locals and tourists alike. And I had to stop at a gelato shop, which was offering delicious, authentic gelato, so refreshing on a hot summer day. We spent only one day in Florence, but it was a day to remember, with its outdoor art museum at Piazza della Signora, the Cathedral, the Vecchio Bridge, and the lively atmosphere created by the Italian people, who gesture when they speak one of the most melodious languages in the world.

A trip to Italy is not complete without a day in Rome. We took a train from the Civitavecchia to Rome, and our first stop was at the Vatican. The lines for St. Peter Basilica were huge, and we did not have much time, so we joined a group of tourists. I had been to the Basilica before while on a business trip to the American Embassy, but this place is worth seeing every time you are in Rome. The entrance immediately grabs the attention with its artistic works, followed by the greatness of the interior, with a vaulted ceiling of the dome, Michelangelo's Pieta, and St. Peter's tomb. I climbed again the 330 steep steps to admire the beauty and the serenity of the place overlooking St. Peter's Square. Then we stopped at the most beautiful fountain in the world, Trevi, and tossed in a coin, which means that one day we will return to Rome. We squeezed in this tight schedule of a one-day trip, a visit to the famous gladiators' Roman Colosseum, to admire the ancient amphitheater with scenes of old gladiators' games. Not far from there was the Roman Forum, which is another ancient Roman structure amidst ruins of government buildings. We raced to the Pantheon, a breathtaking building with large granite columns and an impressive dome, which is a former Roman temple and a Catholic church since 609 AD. A visit to Rome requires a visit to the Spanish Steps, which start at the Piazza di Spagna and end at Pincio Hill. The multitude of people of all nationalities added to my festive mood. We strolled past boutiques of fashionable clothes and shoes to reach the steps and walked up to the top of the hill, from where we admired the spectacular view of the place full of life and joy. A woman cannot leave Rome without new shoes, and I ended up buying a pair of gorgeous green sandals.

There is a saying, "See Venice and die," and my curiosity took me to the city of the legendary gondolas while on another cruise with Royal Caribbean. The cruise started from Venice, and we arrived a couple of days earlier to view this one-of-a-kind city of the world. We landed at Venice airport in mid-morning and were thrilled to find out that we could use a water bus to reach the city. It was chaotic at first when we had to figure out which line of water bus to take, added to the fact that the place was packed with people. A very nice young woman met us when we arrived at the Grand Canal and took us to the apartment, which I booked the previous day. We followed her on narrow alleys and streets and reached an old, attractive building, which was centrally located and close to Piazzo San Marco. It was Mitt's birthday, and we had a special dinner by the incredible Grand Canal, followed by a gondola ride. I was so happy to see sights I read about in the tourist brochures, such as the Bridge of Sighs. This was the place where prisoners in the past paused to sigh and say goodbye to Venice before being executed or transported across the canal to the underground cells of the Doge's Palace. We were out early on the next morning and encountered a very joyous sight of gondolas with gondoliers singing "Oh Sole Mio" while skillfully navigating through the Venice canals. We followed a list of recommended must-see places and visited the remarkable St. Mark Basilica at St. Mark's square. It was a grandiose building with an austere look and elegance, which we immediately spotted as we approached the square. An authentic Italian cappuccino was in order at that amazing place boasting with life and splendor. As we sipped coffee, we enjoyed the scene of happy people passing by, laughing and talking in animation. We continued our walk and managed to squeeze in time to view the St. Mark Basilica, which was another exquisite architectural building dating from the 9th century AD with impressive columns and mosaics. Inside, its Byzantine altar is covered in gold, and there are four gilded bronze horses representing the triumphal four-horse carriage used for chariot racing. It is difficult to describe all the details of the artwork on the exterior and on the doomed ceiling in the interior of the Basilica. We also walked on Ponte di Rialto, the bridge that we saw from the gondola on the previous night, which was impressive in the sunlight just as it was at night. Its peculiar structure of beautiful, artistic design in a reverse V shape with arched openings drew my attention immediately. There were shops with souvenirs and gorgeous jewelry, which could satisfy the desires of the most capricious women.

We were running out of time, so we hopped on a Vaporetto, which is the water transport in Venice, to return to the apartment. I was deeply in thought the next day on our way to the ship as I reflected on the incredible and extraordinary experience I had in Venice, the City of Love, with its amazing channels, ancient architecture, delicious food, and passionate people. While wandering the streets in Venice I was particularly impressed with the displays of Carnaval masks in the windows of several shops. I had not seen any masks as artistic and beautiful in my life.

Another port city on this cruise was Dubrovnik in Croatia by the Adriatic Sea. We had only a few hours to spare, so we headed to the fortress, which encircled Old Town, and walked for a couple of hours, admiring the view of the sea and the town below us. I knew the city had a lot to offer, but we had limited time, and I was happy to have *kevapcica* and beer at an outdoor restaurant close to the ship. This meal brought memories of my student life in Belgrade when this was often my dinner. Spending a few hours in Dubrovnik, a resort town rich in history and culture, impressed me so much that I knew that I would love to return to it one day.

CHAPTER 15
Israel

Israel, the most sacred place on earth, was always one of my most desired destinations. It was summertime when Mitt and I decided to make this trip become a reality. We contacted a tourist agency in Sofia Bulgaria, and a week later we were on a plane to Tel Aviv, which was a direct two-and-a-half-hour flight from Sofia. We like using public transportation, and when we arrived at the airport in Tel Aviv, we looked for a bus. It was very strange that the people who we stopped to ask for information did not speak English. We used gestures to locate a bus traveling towards the coast, and by mistake got off at a stop not entirely close to the hotel. But it was all right, as we needed the walk after the flight. The Renaissance Hotel by Marriott was on the beach and had excellent service. Our room had a view of the sea with a balcony, and we could see in the distance Jaffa Old City with the Jaffa Clock Tower on a hill. We immediately decided that we were going there for dinner. We took a bus for a few stops and then decided to get off it and walk the rest of the way on the beach. I was excited to enter the city as I knew about its rich history. Much of the city was destroyed and replaced with eateries, art galleries, and shops, but it still had an ancient look with its cobblestone streets. It was crowded with local people and tourists, and it was not easy to find a place to eat. We finally found a restaurant off the main area, where we could have authentic Jewish dishes. It was getting late, and we could not do a lot of sightseeing, but we succeeded to stop by and view from outside St. Peter's Church, a mosque, and a synagogue.

The next day was exciting, as we packed for a trip to Jerusalem. After big discussions at the ticket counter at the bus station, we managed to get on the right bus and arrived safely in Jerusalem. Our hotel was within a short walk to all major attractions. The receptionist was very polite and provided us with a map, on which she pointed out places which we had to see. We did not waste any time and headed out immediately after checking in. We reached the Fortress Antonia and passed the Lions Gate in the Muslim quarter on a road leading to the Church of the Holy Sepulcher. I kept looking around and felt a divine love and peace. We stopped at each one of the fourteen stations where Jesus rested on the day of his crucifixion and said a little prayer. I trembled when I saw Via Dolorosa with the last five stations, where he marked his Passions. There were stores selling souvenirs, and we bought a dozen small icons for family and friends before entering the church of the Holy Sepulchre. Inside it was very crowded, with long lines to see Jesus's tomb, the place he was crucified, and the area where he was laid down before his burial. Three denominations shared the church, Roman Catholic, Greek Orthodox, and Armenian Apostolic. The tomb was enclosed, and a priest allowed only one person or family to enter at the time. Our turn came, and I took out the icons. I spread them on the tomb and said the prayer "Our Father Who is in Heaven." I felt a wave of emotions which filled me with sorrow and at the same time with joy that I was at Jesus's burial site. When I walked out, I spotted a group of people with icons bent over a rectangular stone, and a woman explained to me that this was where Jesus was laid when they took him down from the cross. The last place where we stopped was Golgotha, a chapel inside the church. We went up the stairs and came to an altar with an opening beneath it. This was the place where Jesus was crucified. The place was very emotional, and I felt deep sorrow when I touched the opening.

We followed our map, and climbed to the Mount of Olives, which offered a spectacular view. There were churches scattered across the hill on a desert terrain. I was particularly impressed with the beautiful gold domes of the Russian church, and the simple-looking Chapel of Ascension where it was believed that Jesus stepped foot for the last time.

Our next stop was at the Western Wall, where I was directed to go to the area for women. I was very excited that I could touch the wall, which I had seen before on television.

Then Mitt wanted to see the Arab section, but there were men at the entrance who stopped him and did not let him in because he was not Muslim.

We had a funny experience on the train from Jerusalem to Tel Aviv. All passengers exited at the airport, and new passengers got on the train. To our surprise, the train headed back to Jerusalem, and arriving in town, it emptied again. We decided not to get off. Soon a group of Israeli army guys boarded the train and walked straight over to us. They were polite and explained that we had to change trains at the airport to arrive in Tel Aviv. Maybe that was a sign that we had to see the outline of the city one more time.

We finally arrived in Tel Aviv and had enough time to have a last swim in the Mediterranean Sea.

Our flight to Sofia was early in the morning, and on arrival I was happy to smell in the air freshly baked banitsa.

CHAPTER 16
A Trip To Hawaii For A Special Occasion

Upon returning from one of my trips, Vanesa called with wonderful news: Dennis and my daughter were renewing their vows at the place they got married before, Kauai, by the same marriage license performers. What was extremely exciting was that they invited me to accompany them on the trip and take part in the ceremony. The thought of spending time with them and the boys (Dennis had three boys from a previous marriage, and adopted my grandson Jorden) made me extremely happy, but being present at such an important event for my daughter made this trip very special. The flight was long, eleven-plus hours, and there was a confusion at first of whether we had to collect our luggage in San Francisco before our connecting flight to Hawaii, but that was resolved soon, and we were on our way to a dream vacation.

Kauai was just as described in travel books, breathtaking, with lush tropical scenery and a blue-colored ocean with fierce crashing waves on the beach, a dream location for surfers. My son-in-law had rented a condominium right by the water so we could admire the beauty of the island from the balcony of the living room or any of the bedrooms. It was still daylight, so we visited the local fruit store. I have never had a better tasting pineapple; it had a completely different sweetness and texture, leaving in the mouth an exquisite taste. We all love the beach, so we walked over to the place designated for swimming. The boys and Dennis were brave and jumped in the water to be met by gigantic waves. They did not stay in long, and coming out on the beach, my son-in-law could not believe that his expensive sunglasses, tightly secured on the back of his head, were missing, but not his hat. We swam at a pool by the condominium and ended the day with a drive to a well-known location on the island to observe the beautiful sunset. Next morning, after a very restful night's sleep, my daughter and I were sitting on the balcony when my son-in-law appeared, carrying dishes with delicious breakfast. This was a very sweet gesture that I will never forget.

The day ahead of us was filled with exhilarating experiences on a private boat cruising along the Napali Coast, a place not reachable by car, as the coast was steep, with high vertical cliffs. Small waterfalls and streams contributed to the immense beauty created by nature. Our first stop was for snorkeling, and as a beginner snorkeler I did not spend much time in the water but enjoyed watching everybody having tremendous fun floating and taking photos. Next was a stop at a very unusual place, as our tour guide took us through a cave opening only to find ourselves in an open to the sky area surrounded by rugged terrain on all sides. "Here is where some of the scenes of the King Kong and Jurassic Park movies were filmed," explained our tour guide.

The next day was the exciting event for the renewal of the marriage vows of Vanesa and Dennis. We all got up early to prepare for the big day. My daughter was wearing a beautiful white dress and Dennis was wearing khaki slacks with a Tommy Bahama Hawaiian shirt, so appropriate for the occasion and the place. The boys were also dressed in khaki dress shorts and button-down elegant shirts, and I chose a silk dress, which was custom made in Bangkok during my stay there a few years ago. The ceremony was performed in the back of our condominium building in a beautiful tropical landscape on a path overlooking the ocean. Vanesa has hired the same officiants—a husband and wife, dressed in traditional Hawaii clothing. It was a very emotional scene watching my daughter and her husband exchange previously blessed wreaths of the beautiful flower lei as a symbol of love, respect, and commitment. The photoshoot was exceptional as the photographer was skillful at taking photos in natural poses. The perfect celebration of this memorable event was to attend a Hawaiian show at a ranch, which started with a delicious dinner, followed by a ride in an open sightseeing vehicle, and observing a roasted pig wrapped in banana leaves in a pit. At the end of the evening we saw the famous hula dance show of Hawaiian women.

The day prior to our departure, my son-in-law surprised us by hiring Hawaiian women to come to the condominium and give us a Hawaiian-style massage while he and the boys went fishing. This was another unforgettable experience as the two women applied on our bodies creams of natural fruit—pineapple, mango, papaya—with coffee grinds, which made us feel very refreshed and relaxed.

It was time to say goodbye to the beautiful Hawaii Island, but we had a few hours to spare, so we drove up a steep road to the Waimea Canyon, known as the Grand Canyon of the Pacific. It was a truly gorgeous scenery of single steep hills with flat tops, valley gorges, and cliffs with red-colored soil.

Kawaii left me with memories of some of the most precious days in my life as I enjoyed the beauty of the wonder of nature called Hawaii Islands in the company of my daughter and her family. What made this trip unforgettable were the smiles and laughter of my daughter, my grandson Jorden, Dennis, and his boys. Watching them happy filled my heart with joy and reminded me of how lucky I was to be surrounded with kids and grandkids.

CHAPTER 17
Enchanting Africa

FROM DUBAI TO CAPE TOWN

Africa is an enchanting continent, because of its wildlife, its beautiful nature of jungles, deserts, equatorial rainforests, and grasslands. Since I was a child, I dreamt of traveling to this magical land and experiencing life in the African wilderness.

That's why I jumped with joy when Mitt retired in September 2015, and said: "I'd like to celebrate by going on a cruise with Oceania from Dubai to Cape Town. What do you say?" We were familiar with Oceania cruise line from a prior trip to French Polynesia and felt comfortable traveling with them because they used smaller ships and offered an outstanding service. There wasn't much to say. Next thing I knew we were at the San Antonio airport. Our flight itinerary was San Antonio to Dubai with a transfer in Dallas. To our dismay all flights to Dallas were cancelled because of a rainstorm. We wasted hours trying to switch to a plane which would allow us to arrive on time to catch the plane to Dubai. By midnight we realized that our only option was to rent a car and drive to Dallas. We already missed our connecting flight and did not want to be further delayed and miss getting on the ship in Dubai.

We both breathed a sigh of relief when, the next morning, we boarded the United Emirates plane and started our incredible adventure. We arrived in Dubai on time to get on the ship and had a moment to take a glimpse at the Dubai airport, which was amazing with not only numerous elegant lounges and restaurants, but it also had a health club and indoor gardens. We rushed out and found a taxi to drive us to the port. I eagerly looked out the window and immediately recognized in the distance the world's tallest building, the Burj Khalifa.

We easily located our ship and soon settled in our stateroom with a balcony. We were familiar with the ship and walked to the restaurant on the outside deck where we had a tasty lobster meal and enjoyed the view of Dubai. That night I slept on the terrace, listening to the sounds of the waves, inhaling the smell of the sea water of the Persian Gulf, and feeling the gentle breeze.

We could recognize in the distance the outline of Abu Dhabi in the early hours of the next morning. We had only a day to visit this remarkable city, and we decided to hop on a sightseeing bus. I was amazed at the extremely modern architecture of the buildings and kept taking photos. I remembered how I had a similar experience when I saw New York City for the first time and could not stop admiring its skyscrapers. The bus stopped briefly at the well-known Zayed Center, a museum which was built in honor of the father of the nation, Sheik Zayed. I was astounded by the architecture of the building with its exterior design. My camera stopped working at the Etihad

Towers, with five buildings that were a stunning sight with changing luminous colors in the sunlight. Then the bus continued past the breath-taking Mangrove National Park, which stretched alongside the coast with mangrove trees and was populated by flamingos and turtles. We got off at the stop Sheik Zayed Grand Mosque, which is a grandiose building with the most unusual architecture, incorporating images of numerous mosque sites with Moorish archways and Arab minarets. It was all white, tremendous, and sparkling in the sunlight, with manicured gardens in the front. I was dazzled by its enormous, beautiful domes, numerous columns, and marble floors. The interior was just as stunning with shining jewel-ornamented columns, crystal chandeliers, and the most expensive and big carpet in the world in one of the prayer rooms.

Fujairah was the next stop, and we decided to join an organized city tour.

Fujairah's museum was humble, with exhibits of coins, weapons, and farming equipment. Fujairah's fort on the other hand was impressive. It resembled a castle, and the guide explained that it was one of the oldest forts in the region. I enjoyed the drive by a market, watching the city wake up with the smells of produce and spices. Women had covered their faces, and I respected their traditions by wearing a long dress with sleeves even on this hot day. Soon we reached Al Bidya Mosque, which was the oldest structure in the United Emirates and was considered a historical mark. We could not see the inside, as it was designated only for prayers. I was curious about the interior, and to my surprise they did let me in, which I assumed was because of the way I was dressed.

The next city on our itinerary was Muscat in Oman. We chose a hop-on, hop-off tour organized by the ship, which allowed us to view the entire city. There was the old town, marked by gated walls around the port, the palace, and the harbor. We stopped at the sultan's palace for a quick photo in front of the golden emblem at the gates that represented the symbol of Oman. The bus continued to Muttrah Souk, which was in a residential area. I love roaming in markets, and this was where we got off the bus. I knew exactly what

I was looking for, a pair of gold earrings with a special design, like the ones I used to have from a previous trip to Istanbul with my daughter. The souks in the Arab world have everything from clothing, house necessities, supplies, spices, and, of course, gorgeous, to artistically designed jewelry. I was satisfied with my purchase and the stroll in the market. We headed to the bus stop and were happy that we did not have to wait long for the bus. I was thrilled when I found out that the next stop was at the beaches. Qurum Beach had cafes and picnic areas with attractive tropical vegetation and palm trees. Bandar Beach was surrounded by cliffs and was a beautiful sight by the water. I love beaches, and this was a perfect way to end our visit to Muscat.

When we returned to the ship, I lay on one of the futons by the pool area, closed my eyes, and envisioned the scenes I saw in the past few days from the remarkable modern architecture in Abu Dhabi to the history in Fujairah, to the exceptional sights of Oman with its spectacular souk, which boasted in gold jewelry, a woman's dream.

We were at sea for a couple of days, and I made use of the exercise room. I participated in the early-morning stretching classes, used the machines with a view of the water, and did laps on the deck. I sipped specialty coffees at the Horizon Bar, which had amazing vistas of sunrise and sunset. I visited the ship's library and read a book, curled up on one of the lounge chairs by the pool. I dipped myself in the whirlpools at dusk. The evenings were special, with sampling and tasting delicious meals, which were prepared by a world-class French chef, and paring them with my favorite French and Italian wines.

On one of the days at sea we had a drill about procedures in case of a pirate attack. Mitt and I were on different floors and people joked by saying that maybe the Somali pirates already took him. My response was that they would not keep him long and would probably offer me money to get him back.

Our next port was Mumbai, which is another magic city in these far-away enchanted lands. Mumbai is made up of seven islands. We chose a couple of trips offered by the ship, a trip to explore religious sites and a night trip. The religious trip was amazing. We visited all the well-known temples in the city, and we dressed in religious attire to participate in religious ceremonies. There were people sitting on the ground and playing musical instruments at the Guruvayur temple. Here we bought wrapped small packages, which we burned for good health and luck. At the Ram temple we dressed in special long clothing and poured water over one of the avatars of Vishnu for cleansing. There was a beautiful view when we drove by the fire temple and Mosque Island.

We had lunch at the Trident Hotel, which was the best restaurant in Mumbai, and it was there that I discovered that I liked Indian food. After lunch we drove by exceptional buildings—the Babulnath temple and St. Thomas Cathedral, the latter being the oldest church in Mumbai. I was amazed at the colorful and attractive structures of all temples. What particularly amused me was the chaotic traffic, with occasional cows crossing the streets.

The night tour was just as exciting. It started at the night market, where the guide instructed us not to stop and shop. Nonetheless I quickly bargained and purchased two dozen colorful bracelets. A special treat was a visit to a theatre where we saw part of a typical Bollywood movie with music and dancing.

The night scenery was spectacular with amazing structures illuminated by the city lights. We saw the Gateway to India, an arch monument commemorating the arrival of King George V, who was the first British monarch to visit India. It is the symbol of India, and it is a place where the locals gather. We drove by the remarkable Art Deco Indian-style building that had round corners, and an upper part, which resembled a rocket taking off straight up in the sky. An impressive apartment building in the center of town belonged to the richest person in India. Further along the tour, I was intrigued by a mosque that looked mysterious in the ocean. The guide explained that it was a landmark and could be accessed only at low tide. The bus proceeded in the night to a majestic sea tower with incredible modern architecture, which I learned was designed by an extremely talented student. My attempt to describe it might not do it justice. It is a funnel-looking structure, wider at the bottom, and at the top, where there is an uneven ring, which curves higher up, and has walking platforms with gardens alongside the edges. The walkway from the shore to the tower was also amazing. It had a semi-curved shape, with two pathways leading to the tower. This description is not complete, because there are a lot of details which are difficult to explain. We drove by the university, which had a luscious green lawn in the front, and ended our night tour with a visit to an upper-scale nightclub, where we had Indian specialty appetizers and drinks.

Early on the next morning we flew to Delhi and from there we drove by bus to Agra to visit the world-famous Taj Mahal. The flight to New Delhi was pleasant and enjoyable as we were treated as special guests. Boarding was very efficient, and the service was excellent. A bus picked us up at Delhi airport and drove by neighborhoods with manicured gardens and impressive buildings. We found out that a lot of the embassies were in this area.

We did not stop in Delhi, as our goal was to reach Agra and see Taj Mahal before dark. The guide pointed out the important sights on the way. The Qutub Minar, the tallest minaret in India, was tucked in the back of a spacious lawn. The Lodi Gardens in the distance had a picturesque triple-domed mosque. The Gurudwara Bangla Sahib was an important place for worship, with its gold dome and flagpole.

The trip to Agra took a few hours. Traffic was heavy and colorful with tuk-tuks, and at the same time interesting as there were unaccompanied cows walking in the middle of the road. The driver took us straight to Taj Manal, which is a stunning structure of priceless beauty, and a testimony of love, honoring the favorite wife of Emperor Shah Jahan, who died in childbirth in 1631. There was a huge line, but we had VIP passes and walked straight through the gate, which the guide explained was built with bricks and covered with red sandstone and inlays of marble. There were inscriptions of the Koran, but there were also beautiful flowery decorations. This gate separated the inner courtyard from the gardens on the grounds.

The Taj Mahal was a dazzling sight. It stood graciously tall in white marble. It was sunset and the building glittered in gold colors. Its reflection in the pool with the alleys of a beautiful garden alongside it made the scene superb and breathtaking. I was so excited and invigorated by the atmosphere that I ran all the way to the building. When I reached it, I stopped for a moment, gazing at it with admiration. There were two mosques on both sides of the mausoleum and every detail was in a perfect architectural harmony. There were monkeys playing and running around, a scene that made me smile. I noticed the river on the right side as I approached the entrance. The place was of unbelievable beauty and charm, with the illuminated-by-the-sun building. I hurried up to see the coffins of the two people who were so deeply in love. The guide warned us that taking photos was not allowed, but one of the guards saw me hesitate and nodded, which was a sign that I could quickly snap a picture. I walked out in awe and touched the walls. I could not believe that I was at this place, which I knew only from travel brochures.

Next stop was at a fort made of red sandstone, which connected to Taj Mahal and the other structures. Here the major attraction was the marble palace, which was smaller in size than the Taj Mahal, but of equal beauty. The guide told us a sad story that Shah Jahal's son, who, thirsty for power, killed all possible heirs to the throne, and imprisoned his father in the fort. The small palace faced the Taj Mahal, and Shah Jahal could view the resting place of his wife only from a distance.

We left the amazing complex and drove through Agra's vibrant streets, busy with crowds of people, tuk-tuks, and cows. It was an incredible sight of women who wore traditional Indian dresses and shops alongside the streets that offered exotic foods and clothing.

The bus stopped in front of the Trident Hotel, which was attractive with its exclusive gardens, fountains, and a central courtyard of red stone to match the rest of the place. We had a delicious Indian meal and attended a show of dancing and singing, which added to the pleasant experience of the day.

It was recommended to see the Taj Mahal at sunrise as well, so we got up extra early to beat the crowds and get another look at the grandiose and beautiful Taj Mahal. This time the mausoleum was bathed by the morning sun in pink colors.

We missed visiting Goa, but the trip to Agra was well worth it. We flew into Mangalore, where we caught up with the ship. On the way we had a fantastic view of the beaches on the Arabian Sea.

The ship arrived in Cochin the next day, and we found a guy with a tuk-tuk to give us a tour of the place. We saw the Chinese fishing nets, but our driver warned us not to approach them too close, because the fishermen were not friendly. We stopped at a public place for washing clothes, which was their version of dry cleaning. There was a big yard with clothes hung up to dry after being washed by hand. We proceeded to St. Francis Church, which is memorable because of Vasco De Gama's tomb. The guy explained that his remains were later taken to Portugal. There was an Indian night at the ship, and the passengers and crew were expected to wear Indian clothes. Our driver took us to a very expensive place, and Mitt's reaction was that he needed to take us to a store where his wife shops. The outfit I chose was stunning, with green pants and a dress, which had beautiful embroidery in red and gold threads.

The Maldives Islands were next on our itinerary, but we could not visit them because there was an assassination attempt to murder the president.

After a couple of days at sea we arrived in Mahe, Seychelles. Seychelles is the playground of the rich and famous and deserves its reputation. Its scenery appeared spectacular, as we approached it and had a closer look at the island with its lush vegetation and a mountain range in the back.

We booked a tour to the botanical garden that was famous for its spectacular tropical flora. I felt intoxicated by the smell of exotic fruits and spices, and I was astounded at the sight of the palm trees with the biggest nut coco de mer, sea coconut. The guide pointed out that the fruit is only on the female trees, and that the male trees have long phallus-like catkins. "The pollination," he added, "is not understood until now, so there is a legend that on stormy nights, the male trees move to make love to the female palms." I discovered that a popular gift item at the shops were necklaces with images of erotic coco de mer, at which Mitt laughed and said that he couldn't see me wearing one. We also saw a blue pigeon and other exotic colorful birds. What impressed me the most on this tour were the giant turtles. I love turtles, and the ones we saw were exceptional and special because of their size.

In the afternoon we walked from the port to Victoria, the capital of Seychelles. The city was small and easy to get around. The clock tower is a replica of the one in London and is the symbol of Seychelles. Close by was a remarkable market, which spread in the air delicious smells of spices and exotic fresh fruits. The houses of stone and wood with colorful facades added to the uniqueness of the place. Shops started to close, and we headed back to the ship.

On the next morning we decided to visit one of the beaches, which is the islands' primary attraction. We grabbed a cab and arrived at Beau Vallon, a beach about four miles from the cruise pier. I immediately fell in love with it. The sand was white, and the water had a clear blue color. On the way back we decided to be adventurous and hopped on a local, old, small bus of green color with open windows and wooden seats. There was a couple from the ship who we recognized and greeted. The bus took off fast and drove close to the edge of the road with shrubs and steep slopes going down to the sea. It was somewhat scary but at the same time exciting.

Mombasa, Kenya, was a port that I was very eager to visit. Ever since I was child, I always wanted to travel to a country in the heart of Africa. We were greeted by a small band, singers, and performers on stilts. It was a very joyous and warm reception which made me feel happy. Buses were lined up, and guides with flags waited for us to direct us in the right direction to embark on our safari journey. The port was huge and full of containers, which made some people nervous. The road was bad, and no matter how careful the driver was he could not avoid the potholes on the road. The scene on both sides of the bus was heartbreaking, with women in shabby clothing and naked kids crawling in the mud, coming out of little shags or boxes, and men were waving at the bus asking for food. One extremely skinny man started to bang on the bus, praying for bread.

Soon we reached a junction to a dirt road that led to the safari at the Tsavo East Park. This part of the road was less bumpy than the main road. The soil had a brick red color with savanna and semi-arid grasslands that could be seen off the road. We boarded safari vehicles with open roofs and started on our journey. The animals, such as giraffes, zebras, and elephants, were at a distance, and everybody jumped and exclaimed when they spotted them with phones and cameras in hand, ready to take photos. There were no lions, rhinos, or leopards, but we were warned that it was not guaranteed to see all animals. We stopped at the reserve and had a typical African lunch. After a short break we headed back the same way we came, hoping to see more animals this time. Soon we reached the main road, which was extremely busy with heavy traffic. Our guide did not talk much, and Mitt asked him if he was a policeman; usually tour guides were talkative. He did not answer, but after an hour of fighting traffic he realized that we would be late for the ship and called in for a police escort. "See, I knew it," exclaimed Mitt jokingly. We barely returned on time and hit the showers to clean up after the dusty trip.

We arrived at the port of Zanzibar on my birthday, November 14th, and were greeted by a band of musicians and women dancers who were dressed in colorful dresses. I was in an excellent mood and joined them. It was so much fun to dance with them their African dance. Our tour bus took us to a beach in Kiwengwa, where the tide was low and we could walk for quite a while without being able to reach the water. Mitt went further in and brought me a birthday present, a starfish. I was pleasantly surprised when we returned to the ship, as our steward had decorated our stateroom with balloons and signs for a happy birthday. He was Bulgarian, and we enjoyed his company a lot. I also had a special dinner at the Italian restaurant with a sumptuous meal and a bottle of exquisite wine.

The island of Madagascar was another place I was very anxious to visit because of its endemic plants and animals like the black lemurs. We had a day at sea, and I picked a book about Madagascar which had photos of unusual succulent plants, beautifully shaped and colorful orchids, unusual baobab trees as well as native plants known to treat cancers etc. It was early in the morning, and I was already standing on the ship's deck with a bag packed for the day when we docked at Nosy Be. The trip we chose this time was a visit to an open-air market, followed by a drive in the countryside to a Ylan-Ylang plantation of very flagrant flowers, which are used for perfumes and oil. Our last stop was a visit to the Sacred tree with a show of native dancing and singing. I was in disbelief that I was at this amazing place. The market was very colorful with a display of exotic fruits, vegetables, flowers, fresh fish that were offered by African women in brightly colored attire and men who invited to try their produce with a smile. From there the bus took us through the jungle to view the famous lemurs lying on branches in the trees, who were not impressed by the noise of our group exclaiming and feverishly taking photos. A brief stop at the flower Ylan plantation had filled the air with the plants' sweet aroma followed by a visit to the very much revered Sacred tree. We were met by the locals, who gave us robes to wear and asked that we take off our shoes to enter a path leading in the Banyan Sacred tree. The place was incredible, as the tree occupied a vast area with huge roots spreading all over the ground. This was a religious site, used for praying and worshipping, and we were instructed to keep silent. We were met outside by a group of young girls and guys dancers, who performed to the sounds of a fascinating African music, typical for the island. The drive back through Hell Ville provided an insight into life on the island. People lived in huts, but also in two-story colorful houses, and there were covered booths with goods for sale lined alongside the streets. There were small cars, tuk-tuks, and people on bikes on the road. It was a very vibrant and lively scene. At this moment I thought how impossible it is to write about the atmosphere in the African places we visited, as words cannot express deep feelings, and neither can provide accurate descriptions or portray the vivid colors of the scenery.

In Maputo, Mozambique, we chose a tour called City, Sun, and Sea, hoping to get an understanding of life in the city and catch a little sun at the sea. First, we drove to the railway station, an impressive building which resembled a summer palace. The central part of the building had a dome with a clock, and the attached buildings had terraces and French windows. We continued to the open market that was stocked with local tropical produce and was a very pleasant sight accompanied by the aroma of the fresh fruits. From here we headed to the Iron House, a very impractical house which was built with iron and obviously not suited for the African climate. The guide explained that the house was constructed in Belgium and was transported and assembled in Mozambique to be a residence for the governor. However, the house was never lived in and served as a gathering place for the locals as well as for visiting artists.

The Natural History Museum is worth mentioning, as it had a huge display of stuffed African animals. The place looked like an immense immobile safari with lions, zebras, hippos, giraffes, and was an unbelievable sight. On our next stop we relaxed at the pool of a hotel and took a walk on the beach. It was a very pleasant way to end a hot day, with waves cooling off our feet.

The skyline of Durban appeared in the distance, as the ship approached in the morning the biggest South African city on the east coast of the African continent. We noticed nets in the water which were there to keep the sharks away. "There are lifeguards whose duty is only to watch out for sharks," added the hospitality director as we were getting off the ship. Our land trip was called "Valley of the Thousand Hills." We drove through the city and took a road up the mountain to reach Phezulu Park. I could not help but notice that the city resembled Detroit, with deserted houses and no one in the streets. "Crime in the city chased people up the hills where they created new neighborhoods," explained the guide. The road was curving up a hill and leading to our destination of an African village. Upon arrival, we walked around a small building and up to a terrace which offered spectacular views of jungle foliage expanding as far as you could see. In the ambiance of such beautiful scenery, we saw a performance of a Zulu marriage ceremony, which started with courting and all details of the traditions for asking the hand of the bride. I was amazed at the music and the vibrant dancing, as well as the colorful clothing typical for such ceremonies. The acting was exceptional, with gestures and display of emotions, which allowed us to follow the sequence of events in the marriage ceremony. Subsequently the guide shared, "In Zulu culture the man has to pay with a cow for the woman he marries, and the richest man in the area paid forty cows for his wives." After the performance we toured the village, and I peeked into one of the circular huts made of thatch grass and other local materials. There was a mat on the dirt floor with benches alongside it. Clay pottery was placed on smaller mats. A woman dressed in traditional African dress was nearby and smiled. I smiled back and waved at her as I left. From there we followed the guide to a snake and crocodile enclosure. I have an enormous fear of big snakes, but I approached the crocodiles, admiring them for their size and strength. It is customary to have tea in this region, even in the heat, and we savored some of their local teas before heading back to the pier.

It was later in the afternoon, and there were already people who strolled along a promenade by the beach. In an hour the place was crowded with families. Some people walked on the sand, others had a picnic or had dinner at restaurants. I was immediately attracted to a street band playing American songs and started to hum to the music. We ended the evening at the beach, where we sat close by the water. I was amused by watching the people around us who had fun with their friends, talking and laughing.

I knew we were approaching Cape Town when I spotted in the distance Table Mountain and the ridge of Lion's Head. Cape Town was the last port on our itinerary, and we were scheduled to spend three days at a hotel with trips to a winery and safari, courtesy of Oceania Cruises. This was the first time I was so far away from Europe or America, and I felt extremely excited and happy. I ran on the upper deck of the ship from one end to the other and took as many photos as I could.

We followed the procedure for disembarking and joined the rest of the passengers for a city tour. First, we walked in the downtown area and

161

reached the gate to the park Company's Garden, dating from the 1650. The gardens were fabulous, with foliage and flowers of exotic beauty that filled the air with delightful scents. The rose garden, the oldest pear tree, and the abundance of old trees contributed to a serene scene of peace and quietness in the middle of the bustling town. From there the bus took us to Signal Hill, a piece of land which expanded from Lion's Head to the sea. I was intrigued by the history of the hill, and the guide explained that it was used to signal the ships about bad weather as well as to alert people in cases of emergency. We almost reached it when our bus caught fire, and we had to wait for another bus. Nonetheless, we were high up enough and close to the hilltop to be able to view the city with distinctly noticeable rich and poor sections, the well-known Green Point soccer stadium, as well as enjoy an incredible sunset. The trip on the next day was to the top of Tabletop Mountain in a revolving cableway, which allowed everybody to view the scenery regardless of where they stood. I remember how I felt my adrenaline rise when I looked straight down and felt like being on an elevator outside a building, only here it was outside a mountain. The trip was unforgettable because of the most unique panoramic view. There were white sandy beaches, with the sea disappearing on the horizon, botanical gardens, and the vibrating city at the foot of the mountain. Back in town we visited one of their famous jewelry stores as Cape Town is a city known for its exclusive diamonds. A lady gave us a tour and presented to us a tanzanite rock, which was much more expensive than diamonds. She offered to put it on top of our hands, and I decided to try it. The rock slightly slipped, which made the woman panic.

The next couple of days we stayed at a hotel from where we went on a couple of extremely exciting and invigorating tours. On the first day we went up the mountain to reach Aquila Private Safari Ranch. I was most certain that I would see here lions and that the animals would be more visible from a shorter distance than the ones in Kenya. We were in open safari jeeps and could observe the whole scenery without standing up. We took off on a dirt road towards a pond and saw elephants playing in the water and providing quite a spectacle. They hopped on each other's back and splashed water like kids. The rhinos were close by and appeared to enjoy themselves, too, by cooling off in the water. A couple of lions sat in the bushes, which made my heartbeat go faster. I jumped up to take their photo and noticed how one of the lions quickly grabbed the hat of one of the passengers, which flew out of the vehicle. Mitt pulled me down and reminded me that the guide warned us not to stand up at all during the entire ride. But I was happy that I fulfilled one of my dreams to be close to lions in the wild. Then the car stopped, and we were told to get out, which was confusing because the guide instructed us at the beginning of the tour not to get off the vehicles at any cost. But that was an exception, and we were treated to champagne and fruit. The rest of the day I exclaimed every time I saw giraffes, zebras, wildebeests, and the black eagle after which the reserve was named.

Our second tour was a visit to a vineyard, which is another attraction not to be missed while in South Africa. The view from the bus was spectacular. We drove by a range of mountains called "Hottentots Holland," with rolling green hills, wildflowers, and valleys with streams. Soon we approached the Winelands, an area known for producing the best South African wines and we arrived at a vineyard, where we learned the process of wine making.

The panorama was superb, with mountains graciously erected in front of the vineyards, which were perfectly arranged and bathing in the sun. Nearby was Stellenbosch, a major university town, which I tremendously enjoyed as the campus atmosphere anywhere in the world always uplifts my spirits. Walking up and down the streets with art exhibits, paintings, and cafes reminded me of Ann Arbor, only here the scenery was exotic.

We had a free day and took a taxi to drive alongside both sides of the Cape Peninsula and to take us to Cape Hope. The scenery of very modern luxury houses overlooking the water was soon replaced with mountain cliffs. The road was curving along the ocean, and beautiful views appeared of small communities by the beach with white sands and blue, clear waters changing their color to dark blue in the distance. Our first stop was at Boulders, known for penguins at the beach. We walked down a path with an enclosure which kept the penguins safe and away from the main road. It was a remarkable sight and an unusual treat, as I always thought that penguins could be found only in cold climates. Here they were, hundreds of them, hopping on the sand, in and out of the water, in groups or alone. They were small compared to what I imagined them to be, and cute, swaying their little bodies while walking on the sand. Nearby there were groups of kids who sunbathed and swam without paying any attention to the penguins. I imagine they were used to sharing the beach. The drive from Boulders to Cape Hope, known as Chapman's Peak Drive, was breathtaking, with views over the sea for as far as you could see and the mountains on the other side that raised straight up to the sky. From there the road continued to an area with sea cliffs of a majestic mountain on one side and the ocean raging below on the other. Soon we arrived at Cape Hope, the most southwestern point of the African continent. I was eager to see how the peninsula ends, with the Indian and Atlantic oceans on both of its sides. The walk up on a path to Cape Point was amusing, with baboons who strolled along or just stayed by the road. It was quite a sight. They didn't mind us as it appeared that they were used to tourists, but I still did not carry food that could attract them. There was a tall lighthouse on the hill which we had to reach to see the spectacular sight of the place where the two oceans meet. It was hot, and I was glad that there was a funicular. A baboon was sitting at the bottom of the funicular, watching the people standing in line as if supervising the entire process. It was a funny sight which made me smile. The view at the top was amazing, where the cold and warm waters of the oceans met at the tip of the peninsula. I observed in an awe this painting of nature, where the raging sea was known to have engulfed ships even in good weather.

We spent the last evening in Cape Town at the Victoria and Alfred waterfront. The place was festive and joyful as if it was New Year. There were African bands playing music and dancers who performed in the street; the restaurants were full of cheerful people, laughing and having a good time, and tourists were happily going in and out of stores. The souvenirs and the exhibits were amazing, with sculptures of African animals. There were colorful paintings of local artists with themes of African life, scenery, and people. The huge yachts docked at the harbor contributed to the festive atmosphere of the place. I knew that this was a typical daily scene, and people here genuinely knew how to enjoy themselves. Our dinner at a restaurant by the water was exquisite. We ordered grilled seafood with fresh ocean fish and a bottle of a famous South African wine. In the morning we said goodbye to our friends who we met on the ship, a lovely couple from Nebraska. The flight back was exhausting in the economy class of the plane from Cape Town to London, with a connection to Washington, DC, and finally a transfer to San Antonio, but the trip was well worth it.

BACK TO AFRICA

From Togo to Cape Town

After experiencing East Africa, I was extremely curious about the west side of the continent, so when Mitt suggested another cruise from Brazil crossing the Atlantic Ocean to Africa and traveling down the west coast to Cape Town, I immediately agreed and started to pack. The cruise was again with Oceania Cruise Line, and started in Barbados, but we decided to arrive a couple of days earlier to make sure that we are on time to board the ship.

My seat on the plane was next to a young woman from Barbados. She was very pleasant, returning from business meetings in the States. At one point the plane, without any warning, sank, and we both grabbed each other's hands. I thought of my family and felt sorry for the young woman with little kids at home. Then it was all right for a while, but the incident occurred again, without any explanation from the crew. We arrived safely, I parted with my lady friend, and Mitt called a taxi. However, when we arrived at the hotel we discovered that our reservations were for a month later, and we had to search for another hotel. Marriott in the center accepted us for one night. That evening we walked out but did not go too far as the beach was not close, and the neighborhood was not good. I am mentioning this experience because I want to share that it is very important to read the details about any bookings online before you pay for them. Sometimes if there is no vacancy, the reservation is moved to other days.

We moved to the only Hilton Hotel on the next day, which had spectacular views of the sea, but was pricey. Nonetheless, we had a good time enjoying the luxurious resort and taking a walk on the beach.

It felt like home when we boarded the Oceania ship, since we were already on a couple of cruises with them, and I even recognized some of the staff.

The first night was fabulous as we settled in our stateroom and sat on the balcony, breathing in the fresh air, and feeling the soft sea breeze.

Our first stop in the morning was at Tobago. We both love marine life and booked a trip on a glass-bottom boat, with a stop for snorkeling and swimming. The boat passed over a beautiful coral garden and stopped at Buccoo's Reef, which is Tobago's largest reef. I was eager to dive in and see the beautiful and colorful fish of the Caribbean. The guys from the boat lowered a rope, and the people who were snorkeling held onto it, but some of them kicked so hard that I decided to swim away from them. At one point Mitt caught up with me and started to push me back. At first, I could not figure out what was going on but then I realized that there was a current which carried me away. From there we headed to a place called Nylon Pool, named by Princess Margaret, which was a lagoon protected by an offshore sandbar. The sand at the bottom was supposed to be very good for the skin. It was shallow, and we could stand touching the bottom, so Mitt dove in and came up with a handful of sand, which I rubbed on my skin. I remember how other people from the boat did the same, and we all laughed and had a good time.

The following day was at sea. I was thrilled to find out that the ship had an artist loft with an art instructor who was a very pleasant young lady with short blond hair. My first painting was a pelican by the beach with mountains in the background. The day went by without even noticing it. I did exercises in the morning, then painted, walked on the deck, and lay in the sun.

The next morning, we arrived at Devil's Island, French Guiana, which is uninhabited island opened by Napoleon as one of the most infamous prisons known to men. Looking at the steep rocky cliffs by the water, it was clear that there was no escape from this place. The guide told us that prisoners were under a free regime and were even provided with land. The island ceased being a prison in 1938 and currently is used as a space center. We took a walk, which was very refreshing, with a breeze coming from the ocean. Especially interesting were the monkeys, who seemed to expect us. A monkey stood up in front of Mitt, begging for food, and grimaced when it realized that we did not have any.

Our next port of entry was Belem, Brazil. The city, referred to as the gateway to the Amazon River, appeared in the early morning mist with beaches and modern buildings. Our choice for a tour was the Guama River Exploration. After a short drive to the river, we boarded smaller boats carrying around thirty to forty passengers, which took us through channels along jungle flora and fauna. We arrived at Combu Island, which is known for the acai plantations, and the person navigating the boat circled around so we could view the life of the local indigenous peoples who lived in houses built on stilts. We got off the boat at Boa Vista Acara and went for a walk in the jungle. It was interesting to hear the guide's information about the different species of trees, fruits, and seeds. At one farm, an old man demonstrated climbing up a coconut tree to the top, which was unbelievable. The guide also picked a big tarantula spider and said that it was not dangerous if you don't move and act nervous, so Mitt had to try it out. When we headed back, it seemed that the water on the Guama River had receded, and the captain on our boat had to be careful maneuvering it to avoid getting stuck. When we returned to the ship, we found out that the second boat with passengers did get stuck and had a hard time getting out. The next morning, we were supposed to dock at Fortaleza, but to our surprise we saw again the shores of Belem. An older guy from the boat that was stuck had a heart attack, and the ship had to return to take him to a hospital in Belem. We missed seeing Fortaleza and its vibrant Futuro Beach, but we managed to get off the ship in the evening and stroll along the waterfront, which had food, drinks, and souvenir stands. The place was crowded with people, there was music, and the atmosphere was very festive.

Recife was the last city that we visited in Brazil before crossing the Atlantic Ocean to reach Africa. It is a place known as the Venice of Brazil, with its waterways, bridges, and small islands. The inside reef created a barrier from the ocean and was a safe swimming area, which gave the city its name. We got off the ship and headed to our tour bus, which took us through the scenic part of the city across old bridges and into the heart of Recife. We saw the Golden Chapel of Baroque design, which is covered in golden leaf and is an amazing religious site of art. We drove past the Governor's mansion, restored churches, and stucco-colored houses, to arrive at Olinda, which is a historical preserved colonial place and declared a UNESCO site. Here we were transferred to vans, which could travel on the narrow cobblestone streets. We were in for a treat when we reached the city's square on a hill with incredible views of the city and the coast. On the way to the cathedral and Misericordia church, we came upon an exhibit of street art and masks. They were so colorful and expressive that I knew that they would be my next painting project. I loved the inside of the church and the cathedral, with the beautiful, colorful Portuguese tile and woodcarving covered with gold leaves. Standing on top of the hill, I viewed the city one last time, then took a deep breath of the fresh sea air and hurried to the jeep.

The next five days were at sea, which I enjoyed as I could paint. I painted the colorful houses on stilts in the Amazon River, with fishing boats and jungle flora. Then I painted the masks which I saw on the hill in Recife by the church and added behind them a map of South America. Looking out the window of the art studio onto the sea inspired me, and I mixed colors of incredible shades in recreating scenes that I saw. I felt tremendous joy when I filled my art book pages with paintings of the trip. But what made me happy was when at the end of the day, I looked at the finished paintings and thought that I did a good job. And I enjoyed the discussions we had with my instructor and the other passengers—painters about our works. There was also a class project. Each one of us had to paint a selected part of a lion's head, and when we combined all the pieces, we had a very colorful abstract big canvas painting. What brought excitement to the ship was the day we crossed the equator. There was a special ceremony on the ship, which was a ritual practiced from ancient times. The personnel from the ship dressed in costumes as King Neptune, his wife, their royal staff, and the shellbacks (Neptune's sons) and stood solemnly on the lower deck by the pool. The Pollywogs, the ones who were crossing the equator for the first time, which were all the passengers, lined up to have buckets of water thrown over their heads to mark the initiation of their crossing the equator to conquer the seas. The performance of the crew was excellent and very entertaining.

We arrived in Lomé, Togo, and were greeted by music and performers on stilts. By that time, after days at sea, we were glad to get off the ship and see new places. We were curious about the voodoo ceremony, so we selected to attend it, with the anticipation of unbelievable experiences. We arrived at the ceremonial place and saw how under the beat of drums, colorful huts in green and red twirled around and moved. A spirit supposedly interfered, and a person appeared from under each one of them after a few circles on the lawn. Local people, also participants in the show, acted as if being in a trance. To me this was an interesting performance and not a religious ritual. We also met chiefs of different tribes, who were solemnly dressed.

The drive through town on the way to the performance and back was very pleasant. I observed how clean and well-structured Lomé was with a circular landscaped Independence Square in the center, wide boulevards lined with colonial buildings, especially the ones from the German colonial era, and the newer buildings of skyscrapers. The guide explained that the Germans, during colonization, created the infrastructure of the country with building roads and establishing a good education system with mandatory school attendance. I was surprised to hear the guide saying that the Togo people are grateful to the Germans for modernizing the country. We

also joined a tour that started with a scenic drive by the coast and by coconut groves, where we watched fishermen at the beach pulling ropes with
nets full of fish. Then we stopped at a fisherman village, which was quite
of an experience. There were beautiful flowers outside the huts, but there
was practically nothing in them. The place which they called a fish factory
had piles of fish with flies all over. But the people were so friendly, they all
had smiles on their faces, and the kids loved the candy that Mitt bought
them. I went to the bus and took out cases of bottled water, which the children grabbed in a split moment. There was no drinking water at this place,
but the kids were dressed properly and looked happy. From there, we
headed to a hotel at Lake Togo for a traditional lunch of meals cooked with
African spices and couscous. Mitt and a couple of other people did not eat
for fear of catching a virus; their loss. Our next experience was also amazing. We passed through the former capital city of Togo, Aneho, to arrive at
Gliddji, a spiritual site. Here we met spiritual leaders and priests of the
Glidji's sacred forest.

Cotonou, a city in Benin, was the next city that we visited.

I was impatiently standing on the deck and looking in the distance
where the outline of the city appeared, with a beach and tall buildings behind it. The name of the city meant "by the river of death." After the reception on the dock by local singing and dancing groups, we headed to the bus
for our next adventure. Looking out the window, I enjoyed the scenery of a
vibrant city with French restaurants and the Saint Michel Boulevard, like
the one in Paris. The drive was scenic, passing by the peppermint-striped
cathedral, an ancient Pont bridge, and a huge market. The city was very
picturesque, nestled between Lake Nokoue and the Atlantic Ocean and divided in two by a lagoon. We had selected to visit the Ganvie Village, which
was built on stilts. The bus dropped us off by a channel, and a motorized
canoe took us across Nokoue Lake. The guide explained how the village
was created. People left the mainland and made homes on stilts to escape
slavery. It was a very poor settlement, but men, women, and children smiled
and waved at us when we passed by their houses. I was curious about the

children and observed them going to school by themselves on old canoes. The guide caught my eye and said that education was important in his country, and that children attended school even in the most remote areas. Not all natives were receptive to being photographed, and hid their faces, which I respected, but I took a photo of a beautiful woman on a canoe, which I painted later. I spent the next day at sea, en route to the island of Sao Tome, painting feverishly images of photos that I took from the village on stilts, such as those of the woman in the lake and a family standing in front of a house with no glass on the windows.

Sao Tome is one of the islands of the African country of Sao Tome and Principe. We did not have an organized tour, so we walked to the market, which was full of life with tables selling African produce, spices, clothing, and music. People talked loudly and women invited those who passed by to buy their goods. We learned on the ship that when vendors tugged their ears, it meant that their goods were excellent. We spotted a couple from the ship; the woman was Chinese and was very pleasant and friendly, as she liked to engage in all ship's activities. I waved at her, and soon the four of us were in a taxi that took us sightseeing to recommended attractions. First, we saw a waterfall, which was tucked in green tropical vegetation, and we took turns taking pictures. We stopped at a chocolate factory and coffee place, from where we headed to the beach strip. Our companions went to have lunch at a local restaurant, whereas we opted to swim the rest of the day. The taxi picked us up in a couple of hours, and everything was all right until we arrived at the port. The driver doubled the fare, which we already negotiated before we hired him. We learned another lesson: we always had to stress details about the trip and the fare, and make sure that the price includes the entire trip for all passengers.

The next city on our itinerary was Walvis Bay, Namibia. We arrived in the morning and viewed the city from the ship, which is located on the edge of the Namid Desert at the mouth of Kuiseb River. The tour bus rolled out from the port and drove on a very well-maintained road alongside modern buildings and houses by the water. Soon we arrived at Namib Park, to see one of the oldest deserts in the world. The desert was on a hill, and if you climb to the top, you will discover a beautiful view. However, soon we found out that it was not easy to walk up the hill as with every step we took, our feet sank in the sand. At one point I started to walk sideways, which seemed to be easier. Unfortunately, we had only an hour and did not make it to the top, but nonetheless, it was a fun experience, especially the part of sliding down. We left the desert and proceeded to the Swakop River Valley and the Moon Landscape. The Moon Landscape resembled a moon surface, which was a spectacular sand-and-rock formation created by erosion when the rains flowed into the river. "Maybe those astronauts were here and thought they were on the moon," jokingly said one of the passengers. We were told not to climb or touch anything, but Mitt had to feel how the ground felt and picked some of the dirt. Afterwards we drove to the Welwitschia Valley, to look at the miraculous welwitschia plant, known to be thousands of years old and named after an Austrian botanist.

We had another day at Walvis Bay, which we decided to spend at the port. After breakfast we walked by the water and reached the pier. There were stores and a restaurant. A group of local people danced to the music of a local band, genuinely happy, hugging and singing. They spoke Afrikaans, which sounded close to the Scandinavian languages. Our friends from the Sao Tome trip joined us for a beer, and we had a lively conversation about our experiences on the trip. As we walked back to the port, I took a few photos of pelicans and birds, which I found to be very attractive.

En route to Cape Town, I had time to paint a scene that impressed me the most—the one of the beaches at Togo, with fishermen lined up, pulling ropes with nets full of fish. I also painted African flowers as South Africa has some of the most unique exotic flowers in the world.

We arrived in Cape Town, and were transferred to the same hotel as on the prior trip. We had the opportunity to participate in the same activities of sightseeing and to enjoy the seafood at Victoria and Alfred Waterfront. Three days later we were on a plane to Zambia to see one of the wonders of the world, Victoria Falls.

CHAPTER 18
Zambia, Zimbabwe, Dubai, And Marrakech

This trip, which followed a cruise in Africa, was self-organized from home, with careful planning for hotel selection and for visiting the most desirable locations within our budget.

It was February 11, 2018, when we arrived at the airport in Livingston, Zambia. I suddenly felt like I was really in Africa as we were free to explore on our own. I looked timidly around me and tried not to cough at passport and customs control as I caught the flu from people on the cruise ship. We arrived in Livingston, a city named after a Scottish explorer who discovered Victoria Falls in 1855 and gave them this name after Queen Victoria. I looked eagerly out the window of the taxi when we drove through the city. It appeared attractive, with houses of colonial era with varied architecture and style. As soon as we left the city, we entered an area with a jungle landscape on both sides of the road. It was a short drive to the Royal Livingston Hotel at Victoria Falls.

I stood at the reception desk, which was in a wide-open area with a view of the pool and, further out, the Zambesi River. My eyes lit up when I saw zebras walking freely on the grounds. We stayed at a very modern villa with a patio which overlooked the park and the river. As soon as we walked in, we dropped our luggage on the floor and ran out the door in anticipation of seeing Victoria Falls before it got late in the day. We walked to the entrance of the Falls, and on the way viewed monkeys and baboons joyfully running, zebras grazing, and impalas roaming around. The animals did not pay attention to us or the other people in the park. They were involved in their own world and provided us with the most incredible entertainment. We could hear the crashing noise of the water at the waterfall, and there were people who sold tapes with its recordings. Entrance to the Falls was free of charge for guests at the hotel, and we hurried along a wooden path with railing to see the amazing sight of the gigantic waterfall. We both had been to Niagara Falls, but this sight was far more impressive and grandiose. We walked down a trail to get to the bottom, and I was happy to spot a bench which I knew I would need to use on the way back as I was still fighting the flu and was not feeling that well. Down by the river, there were African kids who played in the water, close to shore, but still, the current must have been strong, and it seemed dangerous. I was continuously taking photos, trying to catch as much as possible of this moment of extreme happiness. We headed back on the trail, and I had to laugh as my bench was occupied by a family of baboons: mama, papa, and two little ones. There could not exist anything more pleasant than being in this world of animals, I thought as I was sipping tea on the patio and watching the monkeys play tag. They seriously played tag, as one monkey chased the others but could not touch them if they jumped on a tree stump, which appeared to be a safe place. In the morning, after a very tasty African-style breakfast, we headed towards the bridge to cross over to Zimbabwe and to see the falls on the other side. I knew I was sick, I could feel it, but I did not say a word as I was enchanted by the world around us. There were guys all over the bridge who sold souvenirs, and we bought figures of two elephants and a rhino. They also offered me to do bungee jumping, at which I laughed. I could never in a million years try something like that. I need to add that they checked our passports on both sides of the bridge. The view of the Victoria Falls on the Zimbabwe side was even more spectacular. We had to wear raincoats as the powerful water created a mist and rain all along the paths. And the scene changed as we continued our walk. The shape of the Falls was different at every angle. No wonder Victoria Falls is called "the smoke that thunders" in the native language, because of its mystic view and thunderous sound. We walked for hours until we were totally exhausted and decided to grab a bite in Zimbabwe. At that time inflation in Zimbabwe was so bad that they were selling millions of the country's notes as souvenirs for five American dollars. We stopped at a fried chicken fastfood place and ordered the usual fried chicken meals at a price comparable to the States. When we returned to the hotel, I noticed an advertisement about safari and river cruises in Botswana. "Let's go on the river cruise, please." My eyes were probably glittering as Mitt responded, "Why not." We booked a river cruise for the next day, and being extremely happy from the experiences of the day, crashed for the night.

I woke up early in big anticipation of the river cruise in Botswana. I knew that this was the place to go if I wanted to see most African animals. The best way to describe my emotions is to say that I felt like singing. After breakfast, without saying a word, we hurried to see the Falls again and stood again motionless in front of the grandeur and majesty of nature in front of our eyes. There was so much power and strength in this mighty water that crashed down with tremendous thunder. It was time to get ready for the river safari trip, so we headed back to the villa. We grabbed one backpack, which was packed with sunscreen, a towel, hats, mosquito repellent, and bottles of water. A black jeep waited for us in front of the lobby, and a very pleasant young African man came out of it, nodded at us, and soon we were on our way. Our driver was very friendly and pointed out parks of the beautiful African jungles that we drove by. He told us that one of the parks was known for rare white rhinos. We reached the Zambezi River, and a boat took us across to Botswana. The man who navigated the boat pointed out the spot where Botswana, Zambia, Zimbabwe, and Namibia have common borders. Another vehicle waited for us on the Botswana side of the river and drove us to a safari resort where we met other tourists. It was only us and an Asian guy who took the river tour, for which I was very happy after all previous trips on the cruise with a lot of people crowding to take a photo at the same time. The rest of the group disappeared towards their open safari vehicles. We were scheduled to take a long trip down the Chobe River. And the adventure began. There were crocodiles out in the sun, and some were in the water. At one spot, a hippopotamus was staring at a crocodile, as if trying to decide whether to take on the crocodile or not, and a small white bird was on the hippopotamus, as if telling the hippo, "Don't do it." I painted this scene, and the painting is hanging on my grandsons' bedroom wall. There were herds of buffaloes on the banks of the river, baboons happily prancing around, and impalas grazing grass. Our boat driver stopped at one place which was close to the riverbank and said: "We will wait here for a while as elephants come to drink water at that spot and at the same time every day." Soon they showed up on top of a sand reef with grass vegetation on both sides. They walked in file towards the water. The first one, I presumed, was the leader; he got in the river first, and all the other elephants followed behind and lined up by him. It was an incredible sight. I shrieked when I first saw them and then remained with my mouth open for the rest of the time, watching them drink and quench their thirst. Then the leader elephant stood up, and all fell in line behind him and headed back to the jungle. This moment was worth a million bucks, I thought to myself, or maybe it was just priceless. The trip back to our hotel in the park was just as enjoyable and invigorating as the one in the morning, and we were happy to catch the last sunrays of the day. We arrived at the villa and cleaned up. I was sipping a cup of tea on the patio, watching with extreme delight the animals in front of me when Mitt came and said: "I have bad news."

This cannot be, was my first thought. *We had a perfect day.*

"We missed our plane to Dubai," continued Mitt. "It is leaving right now." I was stupefied. Of course, I was not feeling well and lost track of the days. We ran to the lobby, and with the help of the receptionist, arranged to switch our flights for the next day and remain in our villa for one more night. It all ended well, and the trip to Botswana was worth any delay in travel.

We had a long layover at the Lusaka airport, and there was no passenger lounge, but the people at the restaurant on the second floor were nice enough to let us stay at the booth where we had lunch. Suddenly, we heard people yelling from downstairs; it sounded more like a fight. I looked over the railing and saw a man arguing with a woman behind the counter, and then other people came and talked, all in quite an aggressive way. At one point the woman sat down and talked to somebody on the phone, then rose again, and the dispute went on and on with no ending to it. I was curious why the police or security did not interfere, so I approached people who were nearby and asked them if they knew what was going on and should we be concerned. "Oh, they are making a movie," one of the women said laughingly. So, we had entertainment while waiting for our plane. It was rather amusing, as the man at one point jumped up on the counter.

We arrived in Dubai early in the morning of February 15, 2018. We were a day late, and the people at the reception desk were more than nice to accommodate us immediately. Our room was ready, and they even included breakfast at no extra cost after we told them our story of missing the plane.

I had not gotten over my flu sickness, and after the flight I could not hear in my right ear at all. Luckily, there was a nurse practitioner at the hotel, and the ear drops that she gave me somewhat seemed to help. Regardless of my concern for my hearing, I still thought of booking excursions and stopped at the courtesy desk. A couple of hours later we were off on our desert safari trip. I knew about safari trips in the African jungle, and I assumed that it was a similar one, only in the desert. I was completely mistaken. We were six people in the SUV, a girl in the front, and the rest of us in the back two rows. The guy took off at high speed and started to spin around. At times the vehicle was tilted and almost overturned. It was a good thing that we did not have lunch. The other two women were screaming, and the men were pale in their faces. Finally, we reached our destination, which looked like a camp in the open. There were tables covered with colorful embroidered tablecloths, typical of the region, arranged around a stage for a show in the evening. It was still early, so we took advantage of the offered camel rides. That was a thrilling experience for which I was prepared as I knew from a previous trip with my daughter Anabelle in Tunisia that the camels rise fast, so you need to hold on. We picked a table in front of the stage and made friends with people around us. There was a couple from Egypt, and I asked them if it was safe to travel to Egypt. They both shook their heads. Dinner was sumptuous and delicious, with barbecued meat, vegetables, and spices of the region. The show started soon thereafter. There was a guy who juggled sticks on fire, then another one performed a dance, twirling in a circle for quite some time. The last act was a belly dance performance. The girl moved graciously and stopped in front of us, pulled Mitt by the shirt, and started to teach him how to move his belly. Of course, I filmed it. Mitt had fun and people around us cheered on.

We decided to tour the city the next day. The first part of the day we spent at the famous Deira Souk for its spices and gold jewelry. The gold souk was full of shops with custom-made gold jewelry which glittered in the daylight, and had extraordinary, beautiful, and artistic designs. I do not wear much jewelry, but that did not stop me from admiring the displays. I did not leave empty handed as I ended up getting a tunic with long sleeves, which had golden woven designs on the front. Then we hopped on an abra boat, which is a traditional wooden boat, to cross the Dubai Creek over to the spice souk. The air at the spice's souk was filled with intoxicating aroma. I love cooking, so I was curious to smell the spices that I did not recognize.

After a brief rest at the hotel, we headed out to the Dubai Mall, which had one of the biggest aquariums that I had ever seen. There were scuba divers who swam with exotic fish, sharks, and stingrays. And in the evening, we saw one of the most spectacular shows of fountains in the world in front of Burj Khalifa, with changing colors and shapes projected on the building. It was extremely crowded, but we managed to squeeze in and get to the front by the water. This was a scene which I will never forget.

We said goodbye to Dubai, but I knew that there was so much more to see in this city. I hope that I will return there one day.

Our flight to Morocco was via Casablanca to Marrakesh. As the plane circled over the city, we could see the desert in the distance and, below us, the yellow houses of the city that were nestled together and looked like matchboxes with their similar roofs and windows. I had booked a hotel close to the famous Jemaa el-Fnaa Square and Marketplace, and our host met us outside the city wall. We followed him as he rushed down narrow cobblestone alleys with stands of all kinds of merchandise. I viewed with interest the traditional Moroccan old houses with walls and big wooden exterior doors. The smell of spices was lingering in the air, mingled with a particularly heavy smell of the city. Soon we arrived at our destination, Hotel Dollar Les Sables. We opened a big wooden door and entered a courtyard that was decorated with antique vases and a fountain built with Arabic tiles. The tables were set for dinner, and we looked forward to our meal, which I ordered when I booked the room. A winding staircase took us to the second floor rooms, with windows looking onto the enclosed inner courtyard. A young lady was shaking sheets out a window. I greeted her, and she responded in French, saying that she and her husband were in Morocco on vacation and would spend the night in Marrakesh before heading to the desert. "But the room stinks badly," she said. Our room had a bad smell too, because of a bad odor coming from the bathroom. I held my nose when I used it and decided to sleep in my clothes. The dinner was tasty as it was a typical Marrakesh meal with veggies and lamb. The spices were from Northern Africa, and the meal was cooked with dates and figs, which gave it a sweetish taste. After the delicious dinner we went out to see the popular huge square. By that time of the day the place was swarmed with people. The restaurants were packed, and the food stands sold baked lamb heads; lamb brain, testicles, hearts; grilled lamb with Moroccan spices; snails; shish kebabs; fish, and fruit drinks. The most spectacular sight were the performances of different acts. There were acrobats, a show with snakes dancing to the sound of music, and a guy who sold teeth. There were monkey handlers and storytellers. I just stood in the middle of all that, amazed at this most in-credible scene, which looked like a movie scene from an ancient Arabic tale. The place was overcrowded, noisy, and festive, judging from the gestures of people around us. We walked the entire length and width of the square and peeked in at absolutely all stalls of food. Mitt talked to the locals, who knew English and seemed very friendly. "Are these real teeth?" Mitt asked the man with the teeth stand, and he responded yes. He sold them to people who needed teeth implants. So weird. The walk back to our hotel led to narrow streets lined by souks on both sides for spices, yarns, clothing, ornamented slippers, leather, bracelets, and tea sets.

On the next day we ventured out to see the 19th-century Bahia Palace. We walked down streets with cafes, tea rooms, and small restaurants until we reached a gate. A long garden path led to the palace. The grand court-yard was paved with marble. It was surrounded by a wooden gallery, which led to numerous rooms of the Ba Ahmed's harem for his favorite women and his concubines. At one end was a grand hall with a decorated ceiling of floral patterns. There were inscriptions in Arabic, geometric patterns, and artistic designs. From there we strolled by the Koutoubia Mosque, which dates from the 11th century. It had a tall minaret, which was visible from all parts of town, but was not accessible for non-Muslims, and we could not enter it.

Our next stop was at the luscious tropical Marjorie Gardens, which had paths and tastefully arranged cacti, ferns, and palm trees. The place belonged to the French painter Majorelle, and later was acquired by Yves Saint Laurent, whose ashes were scattered in the garden after his death in 2008. I did not feel like returning to the hotel, so I lay down on the benches in the garden and enjoyed the beauty of the place. We had a very nice meal at a nearby restaurant and continued our tour with a visit to a leather tan-nery, where we observed the whole process of preparing leather for sale. They soaked the skins, after which they squeezed them and put them out to dry. It was a smelly place but worth seeing, according to Mitt. Back at the hotel I walked up to the terrace on the third floor which had lounge chairs. The women from the hotel washed there the laundry and hung it out to dry. I did not feel like going to the room, so I sat in one of the lounge chairs, enjoying the sun and the tranquility of the place. Mitt went out to roam the narrow streets with souks and to check out the square again. We left the next day and arrived in Madrid later in the afternoon. We stayed at Hilton by the airport, and I was so happy to be in a room with normal bathroom that I walked straight to the shower, not even undressing.

I was so grateful for the nice-smelling room, the comfortable bed, and the delicious Spanish breakfast, before we flew back to our home in the States.

CHAPTER 19
Exotic Asia

SHANGHAI, CHINA

There is an advertisement about travel to Malaysia, that Malaysia is truly Asia, but I will start my story with a trip from China to Thailand and Burma.

This was my first cruise on *Star Clippers*, a ship with sails and a very informal atmosphere, with wooden decks, no casinos, and only basic accommodations. There were lounge chairs on the upper deck where the sails were put up and down, and on the lower level there was an area for morning exercises. The cabins were small, with windows and bathrooms with shower, and the dining room was straight down the hall from our stateroom. But I am getting ahead of myself. On the way to the cruise, which started in Phuket, Thailand, we decided to stop in Shanghai. We did not have a visa, but we found out that tourists can spend seventy-two hours in China without visas. However, when we arrived at the airport in Shanghai, we were told that because of a connecting flight in another Chinese town, we needed a visa. An official accompanied Mitt to an ATM machine, and we obtained visas without a problem. It was late at night when the taxi drove us through the sleepy city, and I noticed from the highway that the city lights were turned off. I figured out that it was because of saving power. Our hotel, which I booked from home, was in the center of the city and across from the oriental Pearl Tower, which is a landmark on the Huangpu River, opposite the Bund, and a favorite area for taking walks. Buildings of various architectural styles, Romanesque, Gothic, Renaissance and Baroque Revival, with Neoclassical and Art Deco, contribute to the fascinating look of this historic district by the waterfront. Our hotel was stylish and clean, with a lavish Chinese-style buffet, enough to fill you up for the day. And the first thing we did as in any other new city was to hop in the morning on a two-decker tour bus. This city was amazing with its brand-new skyscrapers and highways. Shanghai expressways have the most impressive and spectacular construction. While on the bus tour we spotted by the expressway numerous bridges with many highways merging from different directions. It was quite a sight. I could not even count all the bridges on it. I was also amazed at the extremely modern new skyscrapers. We were told that the speedy building of skyscrapers in China was because instead of building brick by brick, they use blocks. We drove by the Shanghai World Financial Shanghai skyscraper, which is a perfect example of an amazing architectural design. The nearby Shanghai Tower, considered the tallest building in China, has a peculiar architecture as it resembles a twisted snake. The bus reached Nanjing Road, a pedestrian street with two parts, east and west. East Nanjing extending from the Bund, had the most luxurious stores of fashion, perfumes, silk, and jewelry. There were also food stores with traditional Chinese food. The bus continued to West Nanjing Road, with its numerous malls, a sight just amazing for a country which had nothing in the past. I remember from old photos how people were on bikes, there were no cars in the streets, and everybody was dressed mostly in grey clothing. When we drove by the malls, I could tell from the window displays that they were well stocked with merchandise and goods from the western world. The Shanghai Center, which was across from the Exhibition Center, had three buildings, with a shopping mall, restaurants, a theatre, the Ritz hotel, apartments, and more. It was a city by itself. On the same street one could also visit Madame Tussaud Shanghai, a well-known name for wax lifelike figures. We did not get off the bus at these stops because we planned to take a long walk in the evening. We continued to the Waibaidu Bridge at the Bund, which is a city landmark over Suzhou Creek. It is an impressive steel structure which stretches to connect both banks of the creek. And further on, at Shanghai Old Street is where we decided to get off the bus and explore this colorful and busy district. We immediately headed to the God Temple, which idolizes three town gods and offers a marvelous view of nine palaces. There were restaurants which offered local traditional dishes, but we were not hungry, so we headed to the Yu Garden. On the way we passed the Great Rockery, with walkways, pavilion, halls, and a pond full of fish. It was a small but remarkable garden which offered the traditional Chinese scenery.

Then we walked over to the Bund, which is the symbol of Shanghai and, compared to Paris, has an attractive promenade by the waterfront. Our sightseeing started with a ride in a tunnel under the water, which took us across to Pearl Tower. We sat in a carriage which zoomed into the tunnel, lit up in bright, electrifying colors of unusual artistic shapes. The sounds of music made me feel as if I traveled in space close to meteors. Once at the top of Pearl Tower, I understood why this is the most important landmark of the city. The tower is an amazing sight, with its peculiar architecture of a multi-layered structure that resembles pearls which drop from the sky and provides the most spectacular view of the city. We could spend an entire day at this extraordinary place, but we decided to limit our visit to the three sightseeing decks. The major one, Space Capsule, offered an exciting and imposing view of the entire city, with its newly built skyscrapers, as well as the Old China area, where modern meets traditional Chinese culture. There was a glass-bottom sightseeing deck, which we did not visit, but I know it is an attraction, and who knows, maybe one day I will return to walk on it.

Back in the street, we looked at the map. We like visiting temples, and we changed two subways to reach the Jade Buddha Temple. I was surprised to find out that the temple was active with monks. What made it unique was that it had symmetrical halls and bright yellow walls. Inside it was a very imposing figure of a white seated Buddha, decorated with jewels inside it. This was an unexpected treat as I did not expect to see that temples survived the severe communist regime in China, which prohibited all kinds of religion. A reclining buddha and three gold-plated Buddhas added to this spectacular scene.

We felt that we saw the most representative parts of the city and headed to Nanjing Street for a leisurely walk and window shopping. Our day ended with an amazingly delicious Chinese meal, and we were both happily surprised when the waiter brought to our table a small American flag.

Not far from Shanghai was the Venice of China, a city called Suzhou, with canals and bridges that resembled those in Venice but had an added flair of Oriental touch. We left early in the morning and caught a fast train, which at a speed of two hundred kilometers an hour arrived in Suzhou in thirty minutes. I was not fully awake when we got off the train and headed to one of their tourist bureaus. A very interesting day was ahead of us as we joined a tour in Chinese language. We did not understand a word of the explanations, but we formed an opinion of the place by the views and sights around us. First, we got on a boat, which traveled on a channel alongside a park where people jogged and exercised. Further down, we saw Chinese houses of traditional style bathed in the early morning sun. Our first stop was at an amazing stone garden, The Lion Forest Garden, where we saw man-made stone hills, which had entrances to caverns and were surrounded by water. There were rocky formations that resembled lions and gave the name of the garden. The pavilions and halls on the grounds of the park were built in Chinese old style, with exquisite workmanship. I kept exclaiming with every step I made of how unbelievable this place was. My next surprise was the beautiful view of the Humble Administrator's Garden, a UNESCO site that boasted unusual glamour with buildings, paths, trees, ponds, and bridges. This place was a poetic expression of a scenery with lush flowers and trees between pavilions and halls of unique specific significance and appearance, like the Fragrance Hall, named after the perfume of the lotus in the pond. It was January, and I remember seeing blossoming plum trees by one of the buildings.

The tour also included a visit to a silk factory where I saw exquisite and fine silk garments in all the show rooms. The last place we saw was a temple, the Temple of Misery, in English, where I observed people praying. We explored the grounds of the temple, where we saw Buddha and impressive statues.

The short visit to Shanghai left me with enough impression to make me feel that I needed to return and explore more of the city and its countryside. Apart from the amazing sights, we were also impressed with the people, who were friendly, and with the delicious and healthy food. I was fascinated by everything I saw, and I felt that I needed to learn more about Chinese culture and customs.

The Star Clippers cruise on the Andaman Sea will follow the visit to Beijing, as I am combining two separate excursions.

BEIJING, CHINA

We organized the trip to Beijing on the internet by ourselves before our second cruise in the Andaman Sea. The hotel I picked was Chinese, had good ratings, the photos looked very nice, but most importantly, it was in a downtown area with stores and restaurants. I wanted to see this city since I was a tax consultant for International Monetary Fund working in Russia in the early 1990s, and my wish finally came true. It was the longest flight I've ever had. It took fourteen hours from Dallas to Beijing, in addition to the hour from San Antonio to Dallas. The couple next to us drank only hot water, which seemed odd to me, but my Chinese was not good enough to hold a conversation. I started to take Chinese lessons a couple of months before our trip. My teacher was a young Chinese woman from our neighborhood, and she taught me some basic vocabulary of introducing myself, asking for directions, and shopping. During the flight, I listened to recorded Chinese lessons; we had three meals, watched movies, and there were still hours before arrival. After the twelfth hour, I started to get fidgety and went to the back of the plane, where I talked to a Chinese woman who was going back home after visiting her daughter in college. She was a doctor but did not work because her husband had a business, and doctors were not paid well in China. She looked at the name of the hotel that I booked in Beijing and assured me that it was in a nice area in the center of the city. I already saw the booming city of Shanghai and was eager to see Beijing in this changed environment. I was surprised that there were no lines at the passport control. We got transit visas for seventy-two hours and were off to our new adventure. Our hotel was located on a pedestrian street in the center of the city, and the taxi dropped us close by it. Naturally, we turned the wrong way, but soon we saw a policeman who, with gestures, directed us how to arrive at the hotel. The Chinese language is so rich, and with more than one word for a hotel, I did not catch the word they used. We checked in and asked for Wi-Fi to google places to see, but guess what? There was no Google, and no Facebook, but luckily, we could text and email. The people at the reception desk were nice enough to print for us information and a map about sightseeing from their Chinese website. We were very curious and excited to be in Beijing, so we went out in subzero temperatures to see how the main street looked like. We had a brisk walk and did some window shopping, from which we saw brand name stores that we recognized with familiar products, and other Chinese stores well supplied with a variety of goods. It was extremely cold, and we returned to the hotel where we had a delicious typical Chinese dinner of tofu, rice, and soups. The restaurant was not busy, and four waitresses waited on us, providing us with exclusive service. And when paying, we discovered that tips were not allowed.

Early on the next morning, we took a cab to go to the place which I wanted to visit for years, the Great Wall of China. Soon we were at the foot of the mountain, and I noticed a small frozen lake nearby. We took a bus and then a lift with a cabin to get to the Mutianyu Wall, which was most popular because of its beautiful scenery. The taxi driver also said that it was an easy hike. We lucked out, as it was sunny and we did not need hats and jackets. The path twisted and turned up the mountain, slightly more elevated at places, with towers along the way that provided a spectacular panoramic view. I was exhilarated by the majestic sights. I breathed in the fresh mountain air, enjoyed the winter sun, and slowly advanced to the top of the first hill. I was determined to reach it, since the hike was not difficult, and only at one point it became somewhat challenging because of the walk up on steep steps. I arrived at the top of the hill, from where I had a plain view of the mountain and the beautiful scenery. There weren't too many tourists at that point, and we decided that it was time to go back. I felt energized by the delightful three-hour hike, and we walked down the mountain at a somewhat fast pace. And now it was time to grab a bite at a Chinese restaurant. We were the only customers, so the people waited hand and foot on us and served us delicious dumplings and soups. Mitt had to prove that he could communicate, so he used the phone translator to talk to the servers.

On the way back to the city, we asked the driver to stop at the Summer Palace. It was getting late in the day, and the temperature dropped considerably. There were people skating and pushing sleds on the frozen lake. We walked alongside the lake and reached the East Gate, which was decorated with colorful paintings under the eaves and had side doors, with three big doors in the middle. At the entrance there were two dragons with balls that symbolized pearls, the jewels that grant wishes. There were numerous halls and pavilions, such as the benevolence and longevity halls, as well as a hall of jade. We walked on the seventeen-arch bridge, where I admired the people who had so much fun doing simple things like flying kites. The winter scene was just as beautiful as the summer scene, which I envisioned with gardens and palaces. We returned to the hotel in an excellent mood and turned in for the night, because we knew that another exciting day was ahead of us in the morning.

We woke up early on the next morning as we were very excited about the upcoming sightseeing that we planned to do. We called room service for coffee. A few minutes later the phone rang, and a voice said: "I am in front of the door, come and get your coffee!" Mitt went out, and there was a robot. He had a hard time extracting the coffee and tea from the robot, and the latter took off. Mitt ran after it, telling it to stop, at which time the robot wrote a message, "I am working, don't bother me." That was funny. The second coffee delivery was successful, and we took photos with the robot to memorize the event. It was twenty degrees below, but we were determined to visit the Forbidden City and the Temple of Heaven. We walked halfway to Tiananmen, the Gate of Heavenly Peace Square, when it became unbearably cold. I was shivering, the shawl over my head and face kept slipping down, and the wind was brutally hitting me in the face. There were no taxis in sight, so a guy gave us a ride for twenty dollars in his private car. The Square was huge, and after a short walk we both had tears in our eyes from the freezing cold. I didn't think I could make it, but I bit my tongue and kept walking. I glanced around us and saw the Great Hall of the People Mao's Mausoleum, and opposite of it the National Museum of China. Even in this cold weather there was a line for tickets to the Forbidden City, and once at the counter, we had to show our passports. The Palace was a magnificent wooden building with columns. It was in red and yellow colors, the latter being symbolic of the emperor's power. Mao's portrait was on the outside wall, and the roofs were tiered, which is typical for Chinese old architecture. The place was surrounded by a high wall with towers at the four corners, where there were doors, with only one open to the public. Once in the complex, we were astounded by the sight of the ancient buildings, palaces, and halls of colorful decorative architecture design in Chinese style. Names of the palaces were very much indicative of the Chinese values in life, which are longevity, honor, happiness, and purity. The halls were big rooms where various ceremonies and activities had been performed in the past. The Hall of Preserving Harmony honored peace and happiness and was used by the emperor to grant titles to the nobility. The hall itself was remarkable with its grandeur and decorative style. There were images of a golden dragon in the eaves, and there was a beautiful painting on the ceiling. The Hall of Central Harmony was an attractive sight, with its pavement of gold bricks, a roof with yellow tiles, and dragon images in the eaves. This was the place where the emperor held big ceremonies. The Hall of Supreme Harmony was unforgettable with its outside architecture and decorative style of extended fences with figures of beasts on top of each stake leading towards the building. Its name suggests that the most important ceremonies were held here, such as weddings, crowning, etc. We spent at least a couple of hours in the halls until we ran out of breath and decided that it was time for our next destination. We were happy to see taxis in front of the Forbidden City. We showed one of the taxi drivers the place where we wanted to go and soon, we arrived at the Temple of Heaven without having to walk and tremble from the numbing cold air. Temple of Heaven was a building of worship for the emperors in the past. It impressed me with its architecture of a circular structure, which narrowed to the top. The building, I understood, was an expression of the relationship of heaven to people. It was late in the afternoon, and we took another cab to the hotel where we decided to finish this memorable day with a feast of the famous Peking duck. The restaurant was close by and very elegant. The waiters were very attentive, and the meal was exquisite. We had goose liver in cherry sauce, soups, and wrapped goose meat in thin tortillas with vegetable and touch of peanut sauce. There was a funny incident back at the hotel when Mitt asked for an apple, and the girl at the reception brought him an Apple tablet. We ended this perfect day with a hot shower to defrost from the cold, and tea brought by our friendly robot.

It was ten degrees Fahrenheit in the morning on our last day in Beijing. We had only a few hours before our flight, but we wanted to see the famous Silk Street. Mitt knew that I wanted so much to have a Chinese silk dress. The breakfast at the hotel's restaurant was delicious. I fixed for us noodle soups with vegetables of my choice, which a lady cooked, and then there were deep fried sticks of bread for the soup, with seaweed and so on. They could not get us a taxi at the hotel, and the receptionist gave us a map and wrote on a piece of paper in Chinese the name of the street and the metro we needed to take. The metro station was a couple of blocks away, but the piercing cold was unbearable. A young guy directed us to the entrance of the metro, which was close to the art museum. I would have loved to visit it, but there was no time, and without Google Maps we did not know about it until now. We had to change two trains, but there were employees at each station who gave us directions, and soon we reached our destination. Sila Street was a market for all kinds of merchandise, not just silk. Mitt helped me choose a beautiful Chinese-style silk dress with a scarf, and we back-tracked to the hotel without a problem. We checked out and thanked the receptionist for their hospitality. On the previous day, they sent us fruit and were very friendly and attentive during our entire stay. We took a taxi to the airport and passed by newly built modern high rises. The city was awake and vibrant in the winter sun. The driver suddenly started to swerve into other lanes as if he was drunk. We offered him water, and he pulled a package of food from his glove compartment, which somewhat revived him. We were very relieved when we arrived at the airport. We checked in for our flight, went through security without a problem, and found a lounge. Here we had lunch and felt refreshed and ready to board the plane as the only passengers who were not Chinese.

I left Beijing with a beautiful silk dress in white and blue, which made me happy, and all the memories of its historic monuments, beautiful sights, nice people, and exquisite food. Our flight was very pleasant, as the attendants were polite and made us feel very comfortable. I mostly slept during the entire six hours before landing in Phuket, where we were met by a young woman, a representative of the cruise ship. She arranged for a transfer to our hotel on the coast named Amari, which was a spectacular resort. Our suite was on a hill overlooking tropical vegetation and the sea beyond it. After the severe cold weather in Beijing, we woke up in paradise where it was warm, with spectacular views and a delightful atmosphere. I could hear the happy chirping of the birds, which made me smile and jump out of bed. We put away our winter clothes and prepared for days full of sun-shine and good times.

THAILAND AND THE ANDAMAN SEA

After a hefty buffet breakfast at the Amari hotel and relaxing at the pool, we headed to the pier where we swam and saw black fish with yellow stripes and blue fish close to the surface. It was a perfect spot for snorkeling, and we decided to return on the next day. We were curious about the city and headed towards Patong Beach, a public beach just down the street from our hotel. There were women who gave cheap massages on the beach, and people were sunbathing and swimming, but the water did not look clear. The stores by the water were not attractive. There were maybe a couple of restaurants that seemed okay, so we returned to the hotel.

We came back to this area in the evening and visited the famous street off Patong Beach with illuminated lights and open bars with blasting loud music. Young girls were dressed in skimpy clothes, and guys tried to lure people to the bars giving sex shows. So, Mitt took me to one. There was no entrance fee, but the beer had a price which Mitt misinterpreted; it had one more zero. The owner was kind enough to let us stay, and there I was, about to see a crazy show of women who performed with their private parts. Thankfully, I did not have my contact lens or glasses, so I did not see all the details.

The next morning was another day in paradise, where we were surrounded by exotic plants and flowers. We snorkeled and lay in the sun. I was in disbelief that such a place exists on earth.

There was a show in the evening which was organized by the cruise ship, and we joined other passengers from the ship to visit an entertainment place called Fantasea. We traveled in a van, and I was mostly amused by the scene of people and animals on their way back home. We saw elephants on the side of the road, and the driver explained that they were working elephants returning from work.

Fantasea looked like old Disneyland, with decorative and festive architectural style of the buildings. They served dinner in a large hall, with buffet stations all along the walls. The show was very entertaining. It was a fairy tale of the Ramayana princess who was abducted by a monkey, and after a war of many years, the king got her back with the help of a friendly ele-phant. I enjoyed tremendously the performance of the elephants who walked in circles, stood on stands, and lifted their feet on a certain count.

The next morning, I opened my eyes and looked towards the sea. There was our beautiful *Star Clippers* sailing ship waiting for us to get on board. I jumped out of bed and gathered our things as fast as I could.

This was our second trip on *Star Clippers* in the Andaman Sea, and I am going to combine the two trips in this reading.

We checked in for a transfer to the ship at the Sea View Hotel, which was a walking distance from Amari. This was my second time on a sailing ship, but I was still as excited as the first time. I went up and down wooden stairs, to explore all the decks and greet the crew and the captain. Then I returned to our cabin, which was small but very functional, with a small round window to look out to the sea. I remember one woman crying out, "This cabin is not big enough for my luggage! Where can I put all my stuff?" After the mandatory drill, we headed to the upper deck with a bot-tle of champagne and watched the sunset while the ship raised its sails and set out to sea at the sounds of the beautiful song "Conquest of Paradise." The scene was electrifying, with the sails up and solemn music breaking the silence while the sea breeze gently brushed my face and the sun dis-appeared behind the horizon. This is how we left every port for the rest of the cruise.

Getting up early in the morning, I was happy to see that there was a morning exercise class on the deck. There was sea sports equipment on board the ship—a kayak boat, small sailboat, and a surfboard. At every new island, two young guys and a gal transported it to the beach. What I truly loved was that this trip was all about snorkeling. After a healthy breakfast and sailing for a couple of hours, we reached Ko Butang Island, also known as Monkey Bay. We got off the tender and headed to the beach area rec-ommended for snorkeling. They warned us not to take anything with us because the monkeys on this island steal everything they see, but I thought that a bag with towels and sunscreen would not be a problem. I was wrong.

We left our belongings on the beach and walked towards the sea. I was about to go in the water when I turned around and saw monkeys approaching our beach bag. I ran back, grabbed a stick, and started to wave it in the air while yelling at them "Shoo!" at which all except one ran away. The monkey watched me carefully and finally took off. A couple from our ship was nearby, and we took turns watching our things while snorkeling and swimming. The rest of the passengers and the sports crew arrived soon, and we joined them. I spent the rest of the day in bliss, admiring the beauty of the island and the amazing colorful fish I saw when we snorkeled. I was also happy to use a paddleboard, which I tried on another cruise in the Caribbean. We returned to the ship late in the afternoon, and after a quick shower, I went on the upper deck. The song started with the raising of the sails, accompanied by a spectacular sunset in yellow and orange colors behind a chain of small islands.

At dinnertime we were invited to the captain's table. I told my story about the monkeys on the beach, and the captain looked at me with a worried expression on his face: "Well, this was not smart. Monkeys are wild animals and could have attacked you but let me tell a story about my wife. She did the same, took her bag to the beach, and the monkeys grabbed it and ran away with it. She was upset because she lost her phone, cigarettes, and make up. So, I told her that the monkeys are probably having fun with her things. One monkey is probably on the phone, another one is smoking, and a third one is putting on makeup. The monkey on the phone is probably calling the other ones about sharing the smokes and the makeup." That was funny, but I also realized how crazy it was of me to chase after monkeys.

We arrived in Penang, Malaysia, early in the morning. There were taxis at the port, and we hired one to take us on an all-day trip to see most of the remarkable sights. Our first stop was at the Thai and Burmese temples. The images of standing and sitting Buddha, dragons, white elephant, fish, and paintings of incredible scenes, where the predominant colors were red and yellow, took me to a land of marvels and fairy tales. The Thai temple was sublime, with big statues of colorful dragons and other mystical figures, as well as with a big reclining Buddha. It was like the one I saw on a trip to Bangkok, which I describe in my book *New Beginnings: From Behind the Iron Curtain to America*.

Our next stop was Penang Hill. We took a train to the top and saw a spectacular view of the city, the waterfront, and the bridge. Last place was Chinatown, which I found attractive, with its old colorful houses, shops, and temples with decorative exteriors and interiors with hanging red lanterns. We returned to the ship, but we still had time, so we returned to the part of Chinatown where houses were on stilts and had names of the first Chinese settlers. We even managed to peek into a couple of other Chinese temples.

Ko Adang Island was another island in paradise, with a long sandy beach of pristine beauty. It had thick tropical vegetation of a forest in the back and blue crystal-clear seawater. I can describe this day as a child who played in the sun. Snorkeling was amazing as I was surrounded by all kinds of fish specimens: angel fish, sergeant, zebra, trumpet to name just a few. I could feel a current, so Mitt swam back to shore with me. Then we went kayaking, and I enjoyed paddling alongside the shore. Lunch was served on the beach, which was barbecue with a variety of side dishes and drinks. After eating, Mitt grabbed a beer and went in the water with fish nibbling at his feet while he was standing. He got a free foot massage which is offered at so many Asian massage parlors.

We spent another splendid day at Ko Rok Nok Island, which had a white sandy beach in a bay with crystal-clear blue water, and a thick jungle-like vegetation in the back. Snorkeling was delightful again as I was surrounded by fish of light blue colors and fish of bigger size. Kayaking was also on the agenda, and I went again on the paddleboard. It was so beautiful that we skipped lunch. We met other tourists on the island who came on another boat and were from the former Soviet Republic. Then a couple from the ship showed us a big lizard that wasn't afraid of people, and we made friends with them. It was such a delightful day, that we did not want it to end so we took the last tender to the ship.

Another day at the sea of marvels started with a very delicious breakfast, which was served with fresh fruits from the island, followed by a stretching exercise on the lower deck.

The ship' s next stop was at the island park Ko Surin, which was comprised of five islands. A tender took us closer to corals with fish, and I was so happy that I was getting better at snorkeling. I was more comfortable with fish swimming around me and experiencing tremendous pleasure of being in incredible surroundings of beautiful corals and underwater sea vegetation. The beach was amazing, with white sand and gorgeous blueish green water. We walked more than once around the island and snorkeled and swam. Then we went kayaking, and I was happy to get on the paddleboard again. Life seemed to be so unreal in this marvelous world of serene beauty and splendor.

Similan Islands were next on the list to visit, with Koh Similan being the most popular among them. It was Chinese New Year, and the Chinese tourists filled the beach fast, arriving in speed boats, but they were very orderly; the beach was crowded, but it wasn't overwhelming as they all stayed together with friends and relatives and did not impose on anybody. This island was also a park and was uninhabited, visited only during the day by tourists. This was the big advantage of being on a sailing ship as we could visit small islands. Koh Similan is known for its unusual bird species and mammals like the flying lemur. When I arrived on shore, I felt like stepping into paradise. My feet were on a white powdery sand, and there was a forest of lush vegetation in the back. A tall rock formation by the water attracted tourists, who climbed it for exercise, to get a better view of the island, or simply because of curiosity. Later, I found out that the Chinese visit this island a lot because of the filming of one of their popular soap operas at this place.

Ko Rok Nok Island was another jewel of beauty belonging to the Ko Lanta National Park, with its powdery sand beach and coral reefs, which, again, left us with unforgettable memories of snorkeling among colorful fish in the clear blue waters of the sea. The beach was at a bay, between two lagoons, and resembling the rest of the islands with an amazing beach of white sand and crystal-clear waters for snorkeling, swimming, playing in the sun by kayaking and paddling on the surfboard. Some of the beautiful colored fish followed me in the water all the way to the shore, and I found that extremely sweet. I guess fish are interested in us humans too.

At Langkawi in Malaysia, a name which means "brown eagle," the one thing that I remember distinctly is the giant eagle statute, the symbol of Langkawi, which is in the square by the water. Its significance is in reference to power, strength, speed, and wealth. It was an exciting day as we rode on local boats by mangrove forests, and then had an authentic Malaysian lunch in an oriental village. After lunch, we took a cable car over a lush rainforest with tropical trees, passed waterfalls, and reached a platform where we were afforded a beautiful view of numerous islands. Next, we proceeded by a van and passed rice paddies to reach Makam Mahsuri. I remember that we visited the tomb of the princess Mahsuri, who was wrongly accused of adultery. She placed a curse on the island for seven generations, and it seemed that because of her curse, tragedies really struck the island for the next seven years.

In Langkawi, we did jungle trekking, which was another marvelous adventure. A van dropped us off at a resort, from where we got off the main road and entered the jungle where we saw lemurs and monkeys in the trees.

I love elephants, like my kids and grandkids, so I jumped immediately at the prospect of visiting an elephant camp where they rescued and took care of elephants. Later, at the camp, we learned that they were not released in the wild as they had no survival skills to live in the wilderness. The boat ride from the sailing ship to shore was long and extremely bumpy. Once on land, we were transferred by bus to a bamboo river rafting station. The raft swiftly passed by amazing scenery of tropical vegetation, and it was refreshing to feel the breeze from the water. Somebody from the group said that there was a boa in one of the trees, which, luckily, I did not see without my contacts. I am sure I would have had a heart attack, as Mitt described it to be big with brown spots. After a very spicy Thai lunch, our guides transferred us by buses to the elephant farm. I felt happy, like a kid, feeding the elephants bananas. At first, I was apprehensive of their trunks, but they were docile and did not make any moves to make me feel uncomfortable. Then local young guys hopped on the backs of the elephants and led them to a pond. We followed them on foot and wondered what they were up to. The elephants were well trained and lifted their feet to help the guys get on and off their backs. We reached a pond, and once by the water, we were invited to go in and give the elephants a bath. I was a little nervous at first as I walked towards the elephant that was assigned to me. He looked at me and our eyes met, but he did not budge. Brushing a couple of elephants in the water was another unforgettable moment.

Our next stop was at a turtle farm where turtles came to shore to lay eggs. The turtles at that farm were of all sizes from tiny to eleven-year-old. This was an amazing day with unbelievable experiences and stories to tell and remember.

Ko Kradan Island is an island that brings back a memory which is worth sharing. After a delicious barbecue on the beach, the crew offered us an experience to remember forever. The sports activity guy took us on a rubber speed boat to a cave in a huge rock formation. They gave us life jackets and explained that we would swim in the dark cave for about 150 meters. Then we would reach an enclosed area surrounded by high rocks with green foliage. I could feel my adrenaline rise, as I started swimming in the dark with a dim light from a flashlight carried by the guide in the front. And once out of the cave, I felt good with a sense of accomplishment that I could manage an activity recommended for better swimmers. It was a truly spectacular place to spend the day, but we were on a tight schedule and headed back.

Our last visit was to Ao Phang Ga Island, with beautiful scenery of a sandy beach with cliffs on both of its sides. This was a place just to admire as it was rocky, and swimming was not that good.

At disembarking we exchanged addresses and hugged our new friends with whom we shared stories of our adventurous lives. A trip like this is so enriching in so many ways. We saw and experienced life in amazing places in nature, we learned about tropical vegetation and animals, we swam with beautiful colorful fish, and we met extraordinary people.

BURMA

We organized the trip to Burma from home by booking on the internet flights and hotels that were close to sightseeing places. The hotels I usually choose are four-star local hotels, very reasonable and with all amenities.

We disembarked in Phuket and took a taxi to the airport to visit another enchanted land, Burma. Burma was not initially on my list of countries to visit, but when I saw a photo of Shwedagon Pagoda Temple in Yangon, which is the most majestic and grandiose structure of a temple imaginable on Earth, I changed my mind. Our hotel was across the People's Park, which is by the fabulous temple. We didn't waste any time, and soon after checking in at the hotel, we rushed through the park, which was a short cut to the temple. I was in disbelief that I was at the entrance of this magnificent place with a statue of a giant white lion with a gold-colored head. The walls were covered with beautiful images with Budha tales. We entered the complex, and my eyes opened wide when I saw the gold-covered huge stupa which held hairs of Buddha. We walked around it and discovered that the building was octagonal and at each corner, there was a shrine with a Buddha image for each day of the week. This is different from the Chinese birth signs as, in Burma, you need to know the day of the week when you were born to find out your birth sign. Mitt and I googled to find out our dates and followed what the Burmese people were doing by pouring water over the Buddha image by the shrine of our birth sign.

I looked at the main, enormous pagoda that shone in the sunlight and its top with diamonds and other precious stones that glowed with the most beautiful colors of orange, purple, and red. It took us two days to peek into all the different halls, pavilions, and smaller pagodas around the main pagoda. I could not enter the Naungdawgyi Pagoda, which was only for men, because Buddha's pieces of hair were originally kept there.

I noticed that people bought gold leaves to place on the Buddha. A tour guide nearby explained that there were sixty tons of gold in the main Shwedagon, which was more than in the country's gold reserve. Most memorable were a pavilion with a nine-meter Buddha in a golden robe, and a prayer hall with an eight-meter-long reclining Buddha, which reminded me of the one in Bangkok.

Both Mitt and I like adventures, so we took the circular local train which travels around the city. That was an unforgettable cultural experience. There were men and women carrying plastic containers full of local produce and cooked food, chicken, and anything else you could possibly imagine. The stop at a food market was the liveliest, with a lot of people getting on and off the train. I was stunned at the poverty I saw on the platform. A woman left her slippers in front of a big carton box and went in, which was, I gathered, her home. The train continued and the scenery outside the window changed to paddy rice fields and villages. A woman who sat next to me was very talkative and friendly, and Mitt said that she liked me because of the way she was looking at me. I am sure she was attracted to us because we looked different and were the only tourists on the train. When we returned to the hotel, the receptionist was very concerned when we told her about our train ride. "This train is not for tourists; how did you find out about it?" We both laughed and said that it was indeed a very enjoyable and colorful trip.

We took a plane from Yangon to Mandalay to continue our adventure in the land of wonders. Our hotel in Mandalay was a wooden, big old boat on the river. The cabin was on the deck and did not have windows, so we kept the door open. It was February, and the weather was fabulous, warm, and very pleasant. I stood on the deck and watched the people on a small boat close by who apparently lived there. It seemed like the men just came from work and bathed in the Irrawaddy River. They looked happy and chatted loudly. In the evening, we went to the night market that was close to the pier and walked around the stalls but did not see anything that caught our eyes.

At dawn, we set off to see the sights and hired a taxi for the day. Our first stop was Mandalay Hill, which overlooked the city and provided an incredible view of the old city walls with stupas, the river, the hills, and a range of mountains in the distance amidst fairy tale buildings of pagodas and monasteries. We were rewarded for climbing the stairs to the hill as we reached an incredibly decorated terrace of the Sutaungpyei Pagoda, with columns glowing in the morning sun. A pagoda called The Two Snakes had images of two snakes, and we saw pilgrims who were praying. There were numerous pagodas and temples along the way to the hill that made me feel like I was in a wonderland. At the very foot of the hill was a stunning sight of KuThoDaw Pagoda, which was surrounded by 729 stupas in a straight line. There was another breathtaking view nearby of Sanda Mui Pagoda, where we saw a big iron Buddha statue and hundreds of shrines with inscribed marble slabs.

Close by was Shwenandaw monastery, which dazzled us with wood carving art portraying scenes of myths on the walls and ceilings of the entire building. On the way to Mandalay palace, we stopped and witnessed an amazing procession of people dressed in colorful clothing and young boys riding on elephants and horses. The taxi driver explained that it was a celebration for sending the young boys to be monks. I was amazed by this unusual parade in an exotic environment and watched every movement of the participants until they disappeared in the distance.

Next stop was Mandalay Palace, which is the last royal palace of the royal family, captured during the Anglo-Burmese War. It is difficult to provide a description of the palace, but I will do my best. The palace is centrally located, with many one-story buildings around it that have different number of spires according to the importance of the place. I overheard a guide say that the Burmese people identify themselves with Mandalay Hill and consider Mandalay Palace as a sign of sovereignty.

Early next morning, while it was still dark, we took a boat to Bagan. It was supposed to be an all-day trip on the river with views of the countryside, villages, and pagodas on the shores. It was a good-size boat, with a cabin and outer deck. It was chilly that early in the day, and they gave us blankets. We sat outside on the deck and admired all the beautiful sights of nature and statues of Buddhas with pagodas. The sun came out, and it became very pleasant as its rays caressed my face and warmed up my body. Everybody on the boat was quiet and in awe of the unusual scenery in silence. Lunch was served at midday, which was a typical Burmese meal of white streamed rice and curry dishes of vegetables and fish. In about eleven hours we arrived in Bagan, which is another miraculous place. Bagan has around two thousand temples and pagodas. and a hot balloon ride is probably the best way to view them, but we preferred to walk and visit up-close the most important sites.

Our hotel was a resort with private luxurious houses in a parklike setting by the river. It had a pool, and an outdoor restaurant where we had breakfast, which was included in the price. Immediately outside the complex were pagodas and huts where local people lived, seemingly extremely poor but happy as I saw them laughing and the kids having fun playing. I woke up in the morning exuberated with joy to start my discovery of the marvelous pagodas in a rural setting. We walked alongside a lot of small pagodas to reach the Golden Palace. The palace was glittering in the sunlight, looking enchanted and mysterious, as if hiding stories of the past. It was the first king of Myanmar who introduced the people to Buddhism, and his capital became the famous city of temples and pagodas. The palace was amazing, with eight wooden buildings of exquisite architecture. There were halls for different occasions such as diplomatic affairs, ceremonies, and meetings. In the center of the royal pavilion was the royal lion-based throne where the king and his queen were honored. I closed my eyes and envisioned the splendor and glamour of life in the Second Burmese Empire. We followed the map with sights of temples and reached the Ananda Temple, which is considered unique because of its structure. It had several terraces from where we reached a small pagoda with an ornated top. The Temple is the house of four standing Buddha images that face the four cardinal directions. A mixture of Burmese and Indian style of architecture, it is the most exquisite expression and demonstration of art. The legend is that the monks who built the temple were killed by the king so that there would be no replica of it. We headed to Narathihapatae Hpaya Temple, and I was again dazzled by its appearance. It did not resemble the other temples as it looked like a monastery with spires. The antiquity of the building was evident from a distance, and what was particularly remarkable for this place were the murals inside the temple. Dhammayangyi Temple was the biggest and largest temple in Bagan. From a distance it appeared as a pyramid with terraces. When we arrived at it, we found out that there were four entrances in a cardinal direction and each one had a Buddha on a pedestal, except one that had two buddhas. This temple also had a legend of atrocities. The king killed every construction worker who left a one-pin distance between the bricks. He also killed one of his wives, who was an Indian princess, and later was vindicated by her father who sent men to assassinate him.

Shwesandaw Pagoda, the tallest pagoda in Bagan, was the next site on the map that we picked to visit. This pagoda was also terraced with a stupa and an umbrella on top like the others. There were stairs on the side which led to each of the terraces, but we were pressed for time and did not climb them. This place was considered very sacred as it was said to have Buddha's hairs.

Scwezigon Pagoda was a Buddha stupa that had a gold leaf-gilded stupa in the middle and was surrounded by smaller shrines and temples. Mitt preferred not to walk around it, but I had to see it from all sides. As I reached the opposite end, I was approached by Burmese women who invited me to a smaller temple, and I understood that they said a prayer for me. Then they pointed at the gold leaves, but I could not buy any as I did not have my purse on me.

We finished the day by visiting Thabbyinnyu Temple, which was the tallest temple in Bagan as opposed to the tallest pagoda, which we saw earlier. This temple was all white on the outside with a tower on it and had a similar top as the others. The terraces had stupa obelisks on bases of their corners. It was a very impressive sight. Overall, I find it impossible to give exact descriptions of any of the structures we saw. On the way back to the hotel we spotted a temple with people on its terraces who admired the sunset. I am afraid of heights, and I was hesitant to climb up, but I made it to the first terrace, and once on it, I was in a bliss watching the beautiful last sunrays that caressed the entire enchanted place with temples and pagodas scattered all over the countryside. It was getting late, and we realized that we were far from the hotel, so we flagged a guy with a cart pulled by horses and hopped on the back of it. It was quite an experience as these were dirt roads with potholes, and we laughed as we remembered our childhood days on the farms in Bulgaria.

Another thrilling experience on this journey was the visit to the volcanic Popa Hill, with a monastery on the top. We found a taxi and soon we were on our way. The road trip was lovely as the drive was in the countryside with farmland and villages typical of the region. The driver stopped and let us out at the entrance of the hill. The place was full of life. Women were dressed in colorful clothing with embroidered blouses and floral head bands. Men wore decorated shirts and skirts, and all wore flip flops. Monkeys roamed freely. There were old cars with luggage on their tops, which the monkeys discovered and ran off with bags of snacks. The locals saw that and chased them with slings. The entire scene was quite amusing. The entrance to the top was guarded by two white statues. Images of thirty-seven spirits from Burmese legends, depicted as human beings in very colorful clothing and head decorations, were at the bottom of the stairs. We started to walk up the 777 steps barefooted to the top where Kalat Monastery dominated the view of the area, with smaller temples and the picturesque town of Popa. There were vendors all along the way who sold souvenirs and gadgets of the region, and all that occurred with monkeys who danced all the way up. I bought a local yellow cream for the face which stopped the sweat, something I needed badly in the heat. A Burmese lady drew a flower on both sides of my cheeks. When finished, she smiled at me and refused to accept any money. The previous day when we wanted to enter one of the temples in Bagan, I was stopped because I wore a tank top, so Mitt bought me a tee shirt, but then for leggings, a woman from the nearby market let me borrow a skirt, and again did not accept any money. What I can say about the Burmese people is that they are very helpful, nice, and friendly.

I was all sweaty, but happy, from the very unusual experience of climbing the steps and being entertained by vendors and monkeys on the way. We arrived at a platform with an amazing view of a scenic panorama with temples. The first thing we came across were golden stupas with good-size bells. We walked in a circle and admired all the beautiful gold stupas and shrines.

Burma left me with a memory resembling a visit to a fairy land with colorful and gold images of statues, temples, and Buddhas, amidst a crowd of people dressed in decorative clothing of bright colors. Elephants and monkeys who roamed the countryside added to the lively scenery in a land of wonders.

JAPAN, TAIWAN, SINGAPORE, AND BALI

We arranged a trip to Japan, Taiwan, Singapore, and Bali by ourselves by booking on the internet flights and hotels. For sightseeing, we picked for each location the recommended ten to twenty places to visit.

We started our journey from Japan and worked our way to Bali.

Japan is a country which attracts and amazes with stories and tales about its culture, ways of life, discipline, exceptional manners, and respect for people. I was curious to experience and view life in this amazing country of ninjas and geishas.

We arrived at Tokyo's airport and looked around for transportation to the city, which was sixty kilometers away. The train seemed to be the fastest, easiest, most convenient, and economic way of transportation. In one hour, we arrived at Shinjuku, Tokyo's famous subway station, which by itself was a cultural experience. I had never seen before such a complicated and with so many lines metro system. It was from here that we planned to take a train to Kyoto in a couple of days. Our hotel was not far, and since we had only carry-on luggage, we started to walk. I looked left and right, and with curiosity, examined the people around me and the signs in Japanese language. I couldn't wait to explore the city, so as soon as we checked in New City Hotel (a Japanese hotel, rarely visited by foreign tourists, with comfortable rooms and Japanese breakfast), I freshened up, and we flew out in the street. We reached the Shinjuku pedestrian district, and I tasted for the first time the Japanese famous noodles. Breakfast in the morning consisted of miso soup, seaweed, fish, etc. After this healthy meal, we bought a subway pass for the day and traveled to Asakusa, the old part of Tokyo. Here we participated in a ceremony at a temple. First, we shook a box for good luck. Then we picked up a stick with a number which told us which little drawer to open and found a note with a description of our luck. And finally, we tied the notes to a wire. The temple was at an open market, with a lot of shops that displayed very appealing oriental goods.

Next stop was at the Imperial Palace, which was a park with a moat and high stone walls. I didn't know much of the current Japanese political system, and now I discovered that there is a kingdom in Japan and the royal family lives in the palace. The palace was closed to the public, but we walked around it and enjoyed the grounds. We followed a list of places to visit and went to Ginza District, where I saw the Sony exhibition and tasted a dessert from the recommended bakery by the old clock of the Waco Tower. From there, we hurried on to a famous shrine to view all kinds of interesting ceremonies. There was a big line, and I observed with curiosity the Japanese women, how they behaved and how they were dressed. I do not know Japanese, but from their gesturing, they appeared to be polite and with good manners. They were all dressed in modern fashionable winter clothes. Alongside the road to the shrine were barrels of sake, which was an amazing sight. We reached the shrine and observed how people bought Hama Yumi replicas with arrows to have luck in the new year; it was Asian New Year.

I was most surprised on this amazing trip with a ride on the bullet train from Tokyo to Kyoto. It was interesting to observe how the conductor opened the door, bowed, and thanked all passengers for taking the train on that day, and how the train left the station at the exact second that it was scheduled to depart. It felt like we were flying at three hundred km/hr. I was hoping to take a photo of Mount Fuji, but I was not successful. A lady told me to hold the camera in front of my face and be ready to push the button as Mount Fuji would appear again. I was extremely happy when I was successful in taking a photo of this spectacular mountain the second time.

Our Kyoto cab driver could not locate our hotel, and after driving for a while, he stopped at a police station to ask for directions. But then again, he had a hard time finding the address. I decided to try the GPS on my phone, which, to my surprise, worked, and showed that the hotel was a five-minute walk from where we were. The place was a small, fully renovated modern building in the center of town. It was still early in the day, so we walked to the Kyoto Imperial Palace, which was enclosed by long walls in a park-like setting. And since again there was no entry to the palace, we headed to the market by the hotel, which was an exhibit of the most colorful and tastefully decorated and arranged food displays. We ate barbecued, very tasty fish on sticks and Japanese dough balls with meat. Then we headed to a very popular part of the city called Giom, where we could see geishas by the riverside. We had a delicious breakfast in the morning at the bakery by the hotel and took a bus to Kiyomizu-dera. We walked past street vendors and took the stairs up to Kiyomizu-dera Temple, from where we admired a breathtaking view of the city. Here we engaged in a Buddha ceremony. We wrote on a piece of paper our wishes and placed it in a barrel with water where the paper melts to make our desires come true. We were ready to return, and at the bottom of the stairs we discovered Gion, which is an area with exquisite food stands and restaurants and old wooden Japanese houses. We looked around and spotted a bus station, from where we hopped on a local bus for the gold temple Kinkakuji. The gold temple was a delightful sight in a beautiful Japanese garden, with two floors that were covered in gold. It was a sunny day, and the reflections in a pond of the temple with trees behind added to the beauty of the scene. Another bus took us to the silver temple, which was an equally dazzling sight. The temple and the beautiful trees and bushes of a Japanese garden were also reflected in a pond, a scene that left me breathless. We strolled in the garden and saw flowers of red berries in the snow. The temple was not covered with silver as a statement of imperfection in art expression. This evening, for the first time we had dinner in a restaurant with a revolving counter which offered the most incredible sushi dishes.

This concluded our visit to Kyoto, and in the morning, we took the shinkansen, bullet train, back to Tokyo. After a quick lunch at Tokyo Station, we took the train to Narita, a town close to the airport, which we later discovered to be a very charming place with a temple, shops, and stalls with food. We checked in at the Hilton Hotel by the airport and went out to get acquainted with the city. At one place I stopped to watch how men skinned eels to make sushi. The street led to a temple where we witnessed a religious ceremony with beating on drums and burning of sticks and papers to reach the gods who fulfill wishes.

We said good-bye to Japan and took a shuttle to the airport from where we flew to Taipei. It was a pleasant close-to-four-hours flight, and we had no trouble taking a taxi at the Taipei airport. Our hotel was close to a night market and not far from the metro station. The city was already awake with busy streets and heavy traffic. I noticed that people used mainly mopeds and motorbikes which made sense. We were ready in no time for our planned sightseeing tour. A hotel shuttle took us to the metro station, and we bought passes for two days. Our first stop was at the Longshan Temple.

I watched with curiosity the people who were engaged in religious ceremonies. One woman came over and handed me five candlesticks. Then she
taught me how to pray with her. I was surprised by this gesture and grateful to this stranger for spending the time to teach me their religious ritual.

I was also amazed by the décor of the temple. The columns were decorated with dragons, images of lions, and snakes. There were flowers and
objects on the back tables for the gods. I stood in awe and admired the
beautiful artistic arrangement that was created out of profound religious
reverence. We were curious to see everything, and we walked in the back
to Snake Alley, which smelled of herbs sold in specialty stores. There were
massage parlors and eateries with local food. Further down the street, we
came across another temple with images of gods with big eyebrows. They
were the gods of justice.

We arrived by the metro at our second destination, which was Chieng
-Kai-shek Memorial. There was a huge square in front of the memorial with
a very impressive building of the national theatre and a concert hall. We
were lucky to arrive on time for the changing of the guards, which is always a very attractive and solemn ceremony.

By then it was time for tea, and we stopped at a traditional tearoom to
experience the Taiwanese tea ritual.

Our day was packed with activities. Next, we took the metro to the famous Taipei 101, which used to be the tallest tower in the world, with stunning architectural perfection and cultural elements. We learned that the
eight floors of the tower meant abundance and wealth. When we walked
in the building even Mitt, who is not a shopper, exclaimed at the view of
the merchandise displayed at the Taipei mall. I remember that I stared at
exhibits with shiny and elegant goods and clothing. The elevator went up
at a speed of five hundred meters per minute, and I felt like I was on a fast
ride at an amusement park. We reached the top and walked all around to
view the densely populated city from all angles.

The last stop of the day was at Confucius temple, which was named
after the philosopher Confucius. The architecture and the appearance of

this temple was simple because it displayed the humble personality of its patron.

We ended this perfect day with a meal at the night market by the hotel where we cooked our own soup with noodles and vegetables.

We woke up early the next morning and headed to the National Museum. As an art lover, I tremendously appreciated the ancient paintings and statues. One of the paintings impressed me a lot. It was a scene of the life of people and animals in an Asian environment. The tearoom on top of the building was an impressive place where I opted to have yellow, and Mitt jasmine, tea. We finished the tea and looked at our schedule. My eyes lit up when I saw that we would go up the mountain on a gondola. The cabin had a glass floor, and we had the entire tropical forest in plain view with its lush trees and vegetation. This was a wonderful getaway from the city. We reached the top and walked on a path from where we could view the city, with the 101 Tower dominating the view. Below us were large and gorgeous tea plantations that were lined up in a perfect order with luscious green leaves. We came across a small temple and enjoyed the scenery in the fresh mountain air.

There was still a lot to see, and we returned to the city. We headed to the pedestrian section, where I soaked up all the atmosphere with the appealing and tastefully arranged stalls and stores. A bite at a Taiwanese restaurant was in order after a long day of exploring and racing from one place to another. I remember that we had very delicious sushi and mackerel dishes with sake wine, which we also bought later at the market to take to the hotel. *What would be the next surprise?* I wondered. Well, it was the biggest underground bookstore with stalls of books that stretched between two metro stops. This was a big thrill for both of us as we love books.

After a delicious breakfast on the next day, we took a decorated train with painted fairy tale characters on its sides to the Beitou Springs. We got off at the last station and followed the map towards a river. It was a short walk alongside the riverbank to the famous thermal valley with its jade-color hot springs pool that created a foggy mist in the air. On our way back

I hoped to find a place where we could dip ourselves in the hot springs, but we did not bring clothes for that occasion.

We took the same colorful train back to the city and came across a temple where they performed wedding ceremonies, Xia Hai City God Temple. This was another magnificent place. There were images of gods painted in a very artistic way, which was believed to protect the people.

Next stop was at Sun-Yat-Sen Memorial, which is a memorial of the Chinese National Father. Its architecture was in Asian style, and the building was amidst beautiful gardens that inspired peace and tranquility. We took our pictures by the statue of Sun Yat-Sen and waited to see the change of the guards. This time the ceremony was in honor of the Father. We spent the rest of the day at leisure. We shopped at the Sogo department store, had a delicious lunch of octopus and fish soup, and stopped at a bakery for yummy pastries. We were traveling south on the next day, so we bought a big travel bag at the night market to pack our winter clothes. At the hotel we drank sake to celebrate the end of our trip in Taiwan.

Our flight to Singapore was only two hours. We did not want to miss a minute in this glamourous city, and as soon as we settled in our Miramar hotel by the canal, we headed out. We spotted a sightseeing bus and hopped on it. I was so exhausted from the race in Taipei to see as much as possible that we went twice around the city. While on the bus, we marked places that we wanted to see. I was amazed by the Flyer, which stood up 135 feet off the ground. It reminded me of how amazed I was when I saw for the first time the Viennese Ferris Wheel in Vienna. But the Flyer was twice its size and provided us with a spectacular view of the Marina Bay, the garden by the bay, the river, Merlion Park, and in the distance, we could see Malaysia and Indonesia.

Our next stop was at Little India. I heard music and was immediately drawn to it. An Indian band played and sang dance songs. Nearby were two temples, which I was curious to peek in. There were men wrapped in sheets performing a religious ritual.

We continued to Arab St., where we had shish kebab and tea for lunch at a Turkish restaurant. There was a mosque down the street, but I could not enter it because I was in a summer dress. I was not disappointed because I saw so many mosques on other trips to Abu Dhabi, Istanbul, and other Middle Eastern cities. We hopped on a bus to Chinatown, which resembled Chinatown neighborhoods in American cities.

It was already dusk, and we headed to Clarke Quay. The place was lit up and provided a spectacular sight of a thriving city life. Restaurants and bars were packed, and people walked in groups by the water. We sat across the quay, watched the crowds, and admired the view of the modern buildings that were in the past warehouses. We strolled back to our hotel, which was close by, and grabbed pizza before retiring for the night.

We had one more day in this marvelous city, and we wanted to spend it in the most memorable way. We decided to visit Sentosa Island by cable car, which was an exhilarating experience of traveling from the mainland to the island in a cabin over the water. The lionfish Merlion statue of 121 feet greeted us when we arrived. The statue is a national icon and a reminder of all the mythical sea creatures. It stood tall and majestic above the surrounding beautiful tropical lush vegetation. We knew that there were famous resorts on the island, but we preferred to take a walk on the trail Sentosa Nature Discovery. We are both nature lovers and enjoyed a lot the beautiful flora after spending a couple of days in the busy city streets. We viewed colorful butterflies, magnificent plants, and various amazing birds. It was so peaceful and calm that I understood why Sentosa means peace and tranquility.

We grabbed a bite at a food court which had Malaysian and Chinese dishes and headed back to the hotel, with one last stop at Clark Quai to admire the sunset.

Our two-hour flight to Bali was early in the morning. I looked so much forward to relaxing on the beach, as I had heard of the famous resorts in this city. Our Hyatt hotel had an amazing park of tropical vegetation, flowers, fountains, and statues along the paths. The beach had white sand and pristine blue water, which was exactly what my achy body needed. I did not want to see any more temples or sights. The drive from the airport to the hotel gave me some idea of how people lived, which I could describe as poor and humble. In the evening we decided to explore the grounds and came across a performance of young women playing on local instruments, which sounded like banging on pots. We joked about it as Mitt said that it gave him a headache, but the headache I had disappeared.

On our second day I rolled all day in the sand and swam. The local people were very friendly, and we talked with them. Mitt bought a few souvenirs, and we learned a few Indonesian words. I wanted to get an idea about their culture, and in the evening, we saw a show with a performance of Bali dancers, who wore colorful costumes and danced to a music created for a Balinese legend.

I left Bali with a very pleasant memory of its extraordinary beaches and tropical vegetation. It is an energizing place with a rich culture that is expressed in so many ways by the people, their dances and music, and their legends.

CHAPTER 20
The Caribbean — Star Clippers

The Caribbean is the jewel of some of the best known beautiful beaches in the world, so I immediately said yes when Mitt suggested a cruise to the islands on the incredible sailing ship *Star Clippers*. We arrived late at the Hilton Hotel in Bridgetown and admired from the balcony of our room the view of the sea. Next morning, we had only a few hours to spend on the beach before boarding the ship. We were familiar with the layout and the routine from our prior trips to the Andaman Sea and headed to the upper deck with a bottle of champagne to listen to the song "Conquest of Heaven" while the sailors were raising the sails. The adventure began early on the next morning at Isla Margarita in Venezuela, where we went on a boat trip on a lagoon by mangrove trees. There were signs of love at every corner, so our tour guide said that this was a place for weddings and for lovers. Further on, we saw beautiful flamingos, and it was an absolute delight to watch them in their natural habitat.

Punta Arenas Beach was our next stop where we had a wonderful time. We swam, sunbathed, and enjoyed the view of the sea. The next day was just as wonderful at Isla Blanquilla, where we relaxed on the beautiful sandy beach under the shade of tropical trees and swam in the crystal-clear waters of the Caribbean.

I had heard of the exotic ABC Islands with beautiful beaches and corals, but now I was so happy that I could experience and enjoy their beauty.

The first island we visited was Willemstad, Curacao. As we approached the port, I saw the unique, colorful houses of Dutch architecture lined alongside the port. We had the entire day to explore, and we arranged for a transfer to a private beach, where we snorkeled and enjoyed the sun on a beautiful sandy beach. I finally had a chance to see the underwater world of the Caribbean, with beautiful colorful fish and amazing corals. On the way back we came across flamingos, and I could not resist getting out of the car and watching them for a while. They did not pay any attention to me, as they were probably used to all the tourists who stop to see them. It was already evening, and the island looked fabulous. It was lit up, and restaurants and shops were buzzing with life. We took a ferry to get across and saw a magnificent floating pedestrian bridge which separates the city into two districts.

Aruba of the ABC islands was another attractive Dutch island. We walked past a tower and a fort by the marina and hopped on a tram which took us to the center of the island. I particularly enjoyed the colorful Dutch houses with steep roofs and wondered about the people who lived in them. Then I noticed that the stores had the latest fashionable clothing and jewelry. The tour operator of the tram was a very friendly and talkative fellow who explained that the official language on the island is Pimiento, which is a mixture of Spanish, English, German, French, and Dutch. He told us about a local van service which we could use to get to Eagle Beach. We did not have towels, but that did not spoil our day. We swam and lay on the sand, which I enjoyed. Somehow, it felt good rolling wet in the sand.

It was time to return, and we decided to walk on the beach and enjoy the beautiful scenery all the way to the port.

We went snorkeling at Bonaire, which is a smaller island than Aruba. The guide on the boat explained everything about snorkeling and safety because the water was choppy, and we had to be careful. He talked about the various beautiful colorful fish that we would encounter, like parrotfish. I had problems with my snorkels as they filled up quickly with water, so I did not go as far as Mitt did with the rest of the group.

Isla de Coche had another gorgeous sandy beach with blue-colored waters. It was a day for swimming and a little shopping. I bought earrings and spent some time under umbrellas, chitchatting with folks from the boat.

Testigo Grande was a small private beach with white sand. There were fishing boats and local people sold chicken and hot dogs. I wished they had fish. We snorkeled here as well, but I stayed close to the beach. There were no colorful fish, but the atmosphere amidst beautiful tropical flora was very enjoyable.

When we arrived in Granada, we booked a trip on a smaller luxury sailboat with ten people from the ship. We sailed alongside the island, and the guide gave us a very good presentation of its history, buildings, and population. Soon we reached a spot for snorkeling, and I was again thrilled to be surrounded by colorful fish that gracefully moved in the water. Back on the boat, we had a party with rum punch in a coconut fruit and danced until the end of the trip. Hog Island was our next stop, and here we were greeted by our hosts who served us the biggest barbecued lobsters. We all toasted to our new friendship and the good times with champagne. We continued the party when we returned to the ship and danced till late in the night.

Our next conquest was Grenadines, where we had an exceptionally memorable beach day in the company of our new friends from South Carolina and Germany. We snorkeled, walked on the beach, and I even managed to stand up on a paddleboard. I was happy with my new conquest, and everybody applauded from the beach. Mitt also joined in the fun and pulled me with a kayak. Back on board, we had another spectacular dinner in the company of the captain.

St. Lucia was the last island that we visited, and we decided to spend the day at the harbor. The yachts we saw were not just enormous but also stylish, as those in movies of the rich and famous. St Lucia is known for the Pitons, which are mountainous volcanic spires, but I preferred to enjoy the view from the ship rather than go on a tour.

We returned to Barbados, which was the last port on the itinerary, and spent another day in paradise surrounded by tropical flora and flowers at a hotel, which was a courtesy of Star Clippers.

Time to say goodbye to the Caribbean with its crystal blue waters, beautiful colorful fish and corals, and its white sandy beaches with charming tropical palm and coconut trees amidst amazing vegetation and flowers.

CHAPTER 21
Latin America

ARGENTINA

Argentina is the country of tango and passion, and I was exceptionally happy when we decided to visit it. In preparation for the trip, we took tango dance lessons and learned a few basic steps. A travel agency organized our itinerary from Buenos Aires to Ushuaia, and soon we were on our way.

Our first stop was Buenos Aires, and I was so happy that our hotel was in the center of the city with a room that overlooked the most popular avenues, 9 de Julio and Corrientes as well as the Obelisk Monument. The latter is a historic monument that was built to celebrate four hundred years of the city's foundation and is considered to be the city's icon. It soars proudly in the sky in the Plaza de la Republica.

We tossed our luggage into the room and rushed out. Across the street was the pedestrian area with restaurants, shops, and street tango performances. I stood for a while at one corner and watched in amazement the swift, graceful moves of a couple dancing to the very solemn and melodious tango music. Mitt had been previously in Buenos Aires and knew exactly the spots that we needed to visit. He took me to Plaza de Mayo to see Casa Rosada, which is the seat of the national government. I was curious about the reason for the color of the building, and now I learned the story behind it. The rose-colored building was a fort in 1594, which was destroyed and replaced with a customs house in the 1800s. An administrative addition to the fort was spared and became a presidential office decorated with beautiful gardens. There are a couple of theories about the reason for the building's pink color. One theory is that the original paint had cow's blood to protect the building from humidity. And the second is that it was supposed to neutralize the differences of the political parties, whose colors were red and white. The plaza is also known for antigovernment, bloody demonstrations. I was curious about the other structures on the plaza. I looked at the travel guide and connected the descriptions with the buildings in front of me. There were the Bank of Argentina with big columns in the front, the revenue office, and El Cabildo Museum, which is an extraordinary white structure with a tower. The House of Culture, which is a museum for the former largest newspaper in Argentina, has a very striking architecture, and close by is the Metropolitan Cathedral, where Pope Francis led Mass as Archbishop of Buenos Aires.

In the following days I walked as in a dream, memorizing all the beautiful places and buildings. I was astounded by the Buenos Aires Opera with its white marble exterior and a mixture of French, German, and Italian architecture. I was able to admire the beauty of the interior in the evening when we saw the opera *Fidelio*, Beethoven's only opera. The singing was in German, with Spanish subtitles displayed above the stage. My German is a little rusty, and I did not wear contacts, but I enjoyed the performance and the story of a girl who disguises herself as a man to visit her husband in prison. The interior was lavish, with marble columns, impressive statues, stained-glass windows, and a giant chandelier in the auditorium. There were seven floors with marvelous paintings on the ceiling and gold balconies. After the performance we walked across to the pedestrian street, which was still lively even at this late hour, and ordered the best cabrito asado in one of the restaurants.

La Boca was a very attractive neighborhood that was located by the port and was distinctive with the brightly painted colorful houses with balconies. Women dressed in provocative dresses offered tourists to take pictures with them, and there were restaurants and souvenir shops. I stood in the middle of the famous Caminito Street and enjoyed the atmosphere that was created to mimic the old days of the place.

A visit to Buenos Aires is not complete without a day at an Argentinian ranch. When we visited La Estancia, I was curious to compare the gauchos to the Texan cowboys. There were performances with horses using bola. Gauchos galloped at high speed to snap a decorative, flowery object hung on a string, which they gifted to the women visitors. We rode horses and took carriage rides, just like in my childhood in Bulgaria's countryside. The highlight of the day was the barbecue, which rivals Texan barbecue, with all local trimmings and homemade bread. At the end of the day, I knew that despite the differences, it was the free spirit that was common for gauchos and cowboys alike.

I admire Eva Peron because of her strong personality, and the love that the Argentinian people have for her, so we visited her grave at Recoleta Cemetery. Her tombstone was remarkable, with her statue and a beautiful inscription by the family mausoleum. But it was rather simple compared to the other grave sites like Admiral Guillermo's, whose tomb was decorated with sea and sailing carvings. Dorrego-Ortiz Basulado's pantheon was imposing, with a sculped virgin and seven branched candelabrums.

In the city of tango, which is the sexiest dance in the world, we had the opportunity to observe a professional performance, which left us breathless with the swift, timely taken steps and passion of the couple. Mitt nudged me to dance after the show, but I felt uneasy after the amazing performance of the couple.

On the way back from the show we had an interesting experience with a taxi driver. When we arrived at the hotel, Mitt paid him, but the man exchanged skillfully the bill with a fake one, which we did not notice. He told Mitt that we paid him with a falsified bill and demanded that we pay him again. We were confused and paid him twice to avoid a scandal. Then we discovered at the hotel that this was a new scam invented recently by taxi drivers.

Our next stop was at Bariloche, which is located at the foot of the Andes. The receptionist at the hotel told us that because of its beauty it is comparable to the resorts in Switzerland.

Our tour was early in the morning. First, we walked by Lake Nahuel Huapi and saw the most beautiful sights of the area. The view was even more captivating from the top of Campanario Hill. My teeth chattered from the cold, but I still enjoyed the scenery around us. We could see in the distance the icebergs of Perito Moreno, the El Trebol lagoon, the peninsula San Pedro, and Victoria Island, with the Arranayes Forest. The tour guide pointed out a resort on the island that was tucked in the forest by the water and explained that famous people stayed there, among them American presidents.

We flew from Bariloche to El Calafate and headed to the amazing Los Glaciares National Park. The sight of the glaciers was spectacular, with changing shades in the sunlight of blue and gold colors. The guide told us that The Perito Moreno was the most visited glacier because it was an advancing glacier. It was huge, tall, and very long, with high peaks. We took a boat because we wanted to take a closer look at it. It was a beautiful, sunny day, and the silence and calmness were occasionally disturbed by the chunks of ice that broke and flowed in the lake.

We returned to the hotel excited from the day's experiences, and I wondered if we could go over to Chile for dinner, but the people at the hotel discouraged us by saying that it was not so close and that there was nothing spectacular to see over there.

Ushuaia, which was our last stop on this Argentinian trip, provided us with unforgettable experiences. As soon as we arrived, we took a walk along the coastal avenue by Beagle Channel, then passed by the port, and the historical Beban House with its unusual architecture of side buildings that were connected to a middle structure with a tower on top. We also walked by a building called the Jail House at the End of the World, which is currently a museum with wax statues of criminals. Before we left on this trip, a lady at the gym said that Tierra del Fuego National Park is a must-see place, because of its beauty beyond description. On the next day we took a bus that drove by snuggled-in-the-cold houses to Susana Mount, at the Fuegian Railway, which was built by prisoners. I was excited to be on this small sightseeing train at the end of the world. There was a loud, sharp whistle, and the train took off towards a thick forest by the Toro Gorge. We arrived at La Macarena Station and the Macarena Waterfall, which was a beautiful sight with the water that rushed down the Del Martial Mountains. We could also see some wooden structures that looked like the houses of the native people in the past. The landscape became wilder in the subzero temperatures. There were thick clusters of beech trees, with trunks covered with moss like old man's beard and Indian bread, and there was an orange fungus, which the indigenous people liked. "There are no indigenous people on this land," the tour guide explained. "When the white men came, they introduced soap to the native people to wash themselves. Until then, the natives covered their bodies with oil to survive the cold. A lot of them died of pneumonia. There is only a one-hundred-year-old woman alive, but she has no offspring, so she is the last living native in the region." Sad story. I continued to look out the window and was amazed to see a green parakeet in the branches. We stopped briefly at the National Park Station, where we saw wetland covered with mosses, Antarctic tundra, and frozen lakes by the majestic Andean Mountain. We continued our trip on the bus, and I admired in amazement the serene winter panorama of Ensanada Bay, with Redonda, the Green and Black Lagoons, and the Estorbo Islands.

Back at the hotel, I thought how incredible it was that I saw Ushuaia, the city at the most southern place on earth and at the end of the world. Earlier in the day we saw a sign with an inscription on it saying that the distance from Alaska to Ushuaia is forty-eight thousand kilometers.

COLUMBIA

The package tour that we bought from Latin Escapes also included a visit to Columbia. We watched documentaries on YouTube before we traveled to learn what to avoid during a trip to Columbia. The warnings were about visits to questionable bars, which were of no concern to us. We flew from Buenos Aires to Bogota, and a representative from the travel agency met us at the airport and transferred us to a hotel located in Zona Rosa. This was the most vibrant area in the city, with upper-scale hotels, restaurants, and shops. We had the afternoon free and decided to go for a walk. We did not go far, but we walked through a park and explored the streets full of lively crowds.

Our sightseeing tour started on the next day with a visit to one of the most famous, attractive places in the city, which was called La Candelaria. Walking in this neighborhood is like taking a step back in time and admiring the colonial architecture of homes alongside cobblestone streets. We reached Bolivar Plaza, with its major historical buildings such as the Prime Cathedral, the Presidential Palace, and the National Capital. I will never forget the visit to the Bolivar's Museum and the story about Bolivar, who was considered a liberator not only for Columbia but for Venezuela and Ecuador as well. First, we walked into a very beautiful garden with flowers and entered the house, which was hiding memories of the stormy and passionate days of Bolivar and Manuela, his lover. The tour guide shared an emotional story of how Manuela saved Bolivar at the San Carlos Palace. There was an attack on his life, and she threw herself between him and the assassins, which gave him time to escape from a window.

I stopped at the cathedral to say a prayer and we continued our tour by visiting the Gold Museum. The place was unique because of the exquisite workmanship of pre-Hispanic gold collections. For us women of particular interest are fine jewelry, and I enjoyed and admired their workmanship and art. On this tour we visited a very unusual salt mine six hundred feet below ground. We descended all the way down and entered tunnels, passing by small chambers representing the stations of Jesus Christ's journey before crucifixion. Next, we reached the cathedral, which was fabulous, with chandeliers and a huge cross from the floor to the ceiling lit up with purple lights. The birth, life, and death of Christ were represented at three chapels inside the cathedral. The one representing the birth of Christ was a scene of the birth and the River Jordan made from salt; the central had massive columns representing the apostles and the Christian faith; and the third chamber was with a representation of the crucifixion. This was an astounding, unexpected, and magnificent sight, as I expected to see a boring salt mine with tunnels. The guide said that the middle chapel is dedicated for weddings, and the bride and groom must find each other before the ceremony to prove that they really belong together.

The last extraordinary sight on the list was Monserate Sanctuary—a church on a hill about ten thousand feet above sea level. We opted to walk and see the sculptures representing the stations of the cross and the chapel of the Virgin of Monserrat. The Basilica had incredible statues from the colonial period, the most important one being the statue of the fallen Lord, representing Jesus falling for the third time on his way to Calvary. At the top of the hill was another surprise of beautiful flowers and a well of wishes, in which we threw a coin as tradition requires for good luck. At that height we encountered a beautiful view of the city. The guide pointed at one of the restaurants just below the sanctuary and said that couples visit this restaurant before marriage, and if they do not get in a fight by the end of their meal, they are meant to be together. *Another interesting story,* I thought to myself.

We ended our visit to Bogota with a splendid dinner recommended by the guide at Andres Carne de Res restaurant. Its unusual colorful décor matched the experience with the delicious dishes.

We both love the sea, so we chose to visit Cartagena next. Our hotel was across from a street on the Caribbean coast, and our room had a balcony with a view of the beach and the water. We immediately headed to the beach and were pleasantly surprised when the concierge stopped traffic for us to cross the street. We also like walking, so we headed towards the old town, realizing soon that it was getting late and impossible to reach it that late in the day.

Next day was reserved for a lesson in history and delightful experiences in touring the city. We headed to the old town, hidden behind walls and fortresses, and were immediately stunned by the beautiful view of old colorful houses from colonial times lined along cobblestone narrow streets. We spotted from a distance the clock tower of colonial era architecture and headed towards it. Then we walked by attractive sights, such as the San Pedro Claver Church of stone exterior, and the art museum. At Plaza Santa Domingo we saw the sculpture of Botero's fat lady. Botero's art is hard to miss with paintings of fat women. The tour guide said that at first, he was not recognized in his country, but became famous after his work became prominent in Europe.

Castillon Felipe is within walking distance of the old town and was on our list to see and learn about the country's colonial history. Besides a place of significant history, which took us back to the days of pirates and English invasion, it was the best location from where we could view the entire city.

On our last day in Colombia, we took a boat ride to the Rosario Islands. I expected to see sandy beaches, but we went to a lagoon with a small swimming area. Mitt and I found canoes and paddled to a nearby strip of land. Mitt went out first, and I followed soon thereafter. It was funny because Mitt did not know until then that I could use a canoe, so, when he saw me, he looked worried and yelled out: "How did you get here?" I pointed at the canoe, and he laughed.

The boat ride on our way back offered beautiful views of Cartagena's beaches and contrasts between the city's modern buildings and the old town.

When we left Columbia, we knew that we only had a glimpse of its beauty and that we needed to return one day for more enriching and wonderful experiences.

PERU AND ECUADOR

Peru always fascinated me from readings about its culture, landscape, history, and, of course, the magnificent Machu Picchu. We booked a trip to Peru and Ecuador, which was organized by the tourist agency Latin Escape. We liked to use their services because the tours they offered were private. We were met at the airport, transferred to hotels, and taken on sightseeing excursions.

Our flight to Lima, Peru, was pleasant and I have a funny story to tell. Next to Mitt sat an older Peruvian woman, who immediately called him gringo. I tried to explain that we were both born in Bulgaria, Europe, but that did not change her mind. "Gringos," she said loudly, and moved to another seat. My intent is not to write extensively about the history of the Spanish conquest of Peru, but it was brutal compared to other countries, like Mexico. It was a night flight, and after being served dinner and drinks, we comfortably relaxed until the smell of the morning coffee.

Our hotel in Lima was in the Miraflores District, a residential and upscale neighborhood close to Kennedy Park and within walking distance to the Pacific Coast. We were excited to explore this new city to us, so, after a quick freshening up, we headed out to Larco Del Mar, which is a unique shopping and entertainment center built on a cliff by the ocean. We were getting hungry, so we ordered the familiar to us dish, paella, at Tantus Restaurant, which was extremely tasty, and then hurried back to the hotel, not to be late for an afternoon sightseeing tour. We left as scheduled in a small van, but by this time of the day, the city was congested with traffic, and it took forever to get to the first plaza, San Martin, and then Plaza Mayor. We visited the catacombs, a train station, the bishop palace, Lima Cathedral with the Christ altar made of solid ivory, the San Francisco convent, and the embassy district in Isidoros. Plaza San Martin was impressive with the Colon Theater, Hotel Bolivar, the Sudamera buildings, all in baroque style. The plaza immediately caught my eye with the monument of San Jose Martin in the middle, with benches and handrails of marble, water fountains, gardens with flowers, and streetlamps of bronze. Plaza Major, by its name, signifies a significant square, and here were magnificent buildings like the cathedral, the government palace, the archbishop's palace, the municipal palace, and Palacio de la Union. The façades of these buildings were mostly of dark yellow color, which is found on most buildings in Peru. The cathedral was what impressed me the most, with its resemblance to the cathedral in Seville. It was grandiose with numerous chapels and had splendid details. We even took a tour of the catacombs, a place with thousands of skulls. We did not visit the interior of any of the palaces. A walk by them was sufficient to tell us a story of the glorified times in them. We were dropped off at Larco Del Mar where we had dinner of whole fish, a very delicious ceviche, and the local popular drink, pisco sour.

The next day was a free day. After breakfast we headed down a steep street that led to the beach, where we sat on rocks and drank guanabana juice. It was Sunday, and they had aerobic exercise and tai chi in Kennedy Park by the hotel, which I gladly joined.

This afternoon we said goodbye to Lima and headed to the airport for our next adventure—a visit to the city of Cusco.

We arrived in Cusco in the evening, and the tour representative took us to the hotel, which was an authentic Peruvian building with stone steps in the front as well as inside which led to our room on the second floor. We had tea from coca leaves, which was interesting, but I learned that all hotels offered such tea because of the altitude, eleven thousand feet. It was dinner time, and we took a walk towards the square on cobblestone streets with historic colonial colorful houses in blue, yellow, and white with blue shutters. I was completely stunned at the view of the main square Plaza d'Armas. There were two magnificent churches, the Cathedral, built of stone from Inka monuments with two chapels on both sides, and Iglesia de la Compania de Jesus. The cathedral itself is a treasure of art and beauty, with paintings of virgins, saints, and statues; it has a huge and magnificent gold leaf plaster. The Iglesia also rivaled in beauty with its splendid architecture and paintings. The buildings around the square were of colonial and Inca styles. We chose a restaurant on the second floor of one of the houses on the square with live Peruvian music and view of the Cathedral. We both sat in silence and tried to absorb the uniqueness of this place. On our way back we were surprised by a torrential rain, which flooded the streets with fast-running water, but we managed to buy rain coats and return safely to the hotel.

On the next day we had our clothes and sneakers dried at the laundromat by the hotel, after which we met our guide and started a tour of the city. I was particularly amazed by the Temple of Sun. The tour guide told us a story of how the use of astrology helped the Inkas determine the seasons for farming, the tilting of the soil, planting, and harvesting. A fence with solid gold on it surrounded the temple, which was in perfect symmetry, and windows of the temple served as a calendar for June 21, a time to work, and December 21, a time to plant. We were told that the Inkas worship three animals: the condor, who is connected to heaven; the puma, which represents strength and wisdom; and the serpent, which has a connection with the earth. The guide explained that the Inkas worshipped and sacrificed the black llama, because there is a black shadow in the Milky Way in the shape of a llama.

Fortress Sacsayhuaman was made up of three terraces built with perfect stones which represented former houses, shrines, towers, roads, with a huge main wall in zigzag. The two tunnels were intriguing, where we saw the Inkas throne made of stone that resembled a bench. It's an archeo-logical site like no other that I've ever seen before because of its perfection and harmony. A short stop at the water temple, built also perfectly with stones, had a story of how priests would bathe there before service.

Machu Picchu was the place that I wanted so much to visit because of its uniqueness, history, and the guide's information that it gives visitors an energy from divine forces. After a three-hour very comfortable train ride, during which I exclaimed at every new scenery alongside the Urubamba River, we reached Agua Calientes. The train was designed to look very fes-tive, and the last stop was at a station in a garden of tropical flowers and vegetation. Agua Calientes is a very attractive town. There is a river that runs through it, with hotels, hostels, and restaurants on both sides and at-tractive cobblestone streets, but what makes it famous is that it is the gate to Machu Picchu. We were transported by bus to the Citadelle, which was at the top of the mountain overlooking a deep canyon formed by the River Urubamba. Here we started our tour of Machu Pichu, the lost city. The guide told us the story of how the Incas fled from Machu Picchu because they were afraid of the Spanish invasion. He explained that an explorer discovered the dwellings in 1911 with the help of a local boy. The complex is a wonder of man's creation, as it provides an impressive sight of being nestled among the high and beautiful peaks of the mountains and forests of various trees that start from the bottom of the Urubamba River. The weather changed, and so did the different colors of sunrays reflected on the slopes of the mountains enveloped in misty fog. There were llamas at the top of the complex that gave a very authentic look of the region. The emperor's quarters could be spotted easily as they were isolated with a staircase that connected them to the plaza below. And close by was the tem-ple of the sun, which had again astrological significance with the sun that shined in June on the temple's windows. Above the plaza, on a platform, stood a massive rock which was believed to have some relation to the sun and the clock. Alongside the plaza were a couple of temples, with broken pieces of pottery alongside the one. The houses looked like they were one-story buildings of stones that fitted exactly without mortar. The perfect terraces that surrounded Machu Picchu demonstrated that there was an excellent drainage system for the planted crops of corn, quinoa, and potatoes. And everything was connected by steps. Looking closer at the complex, it was easy to distinguish the different districts that started with the most obvious ones from the terraced land. Across from the emperor's place were the houses of the rest of the people, which were not built so perfectly. And there was a city wall for protection and security. I cannot say that I felt some extraordinary power, but I recognized the beauty of the place. I remembered how I was spiritually and emotionally charged when I visited the Rodopi, Pirin, and Rila Mountains in Bulgaria, and the Colorado and the Smoky Mountains in America, as these are the places close to my heart, my homeland in Bulgaria, and America, my second home where I found freedom and happiness.

A train took us back to Cusco, and we took another last walk in this amazing place with beautiful music, history, and amazing architecture. As we approached the center, we heard lively music and indigenous peoples dressed in bright colored outfits danced down the street. I wanted to join them, but before I did, I asked a woman about the event, and she said that it was a demonstration against a decision of the local government to build on indigenous land. This changed my mind about dancing with them as I did not want to be a part of a political demonstration in a foreign land.

We had our customary coca tea, and soon our guide arrived to take us to a bus to continue our tour to our next destination. The ride from Cusco to Puno took ten hours, with stops every now and then so that we could get used to the increase in altitude. Soon we stopped on the road at a spot of 4,300 meters, from where we could see mountain peaks covered in snow, and from where the River Urubamba originated. On our way further on, we visited a village with a church of eclectic style that had a combination of the Catholic, Inca, and Moor images. The Raqchi archeological site was another wonder of Inkas civilization, with traces of buildings perceived to be religious. We saw barracks for the army and numerous circular buildings thought to be former stores. Here we bought some souvenirs and visited the Temple of God, which was dedicated to the supreme Inka God.

We arrived in Puno late in the afternoon and stopped at a pharmacy for Mitt's diarrhea sickness. For readers' information, the drug called Giardia Lamblia is the best medication Diarin for turista. We had soup for dinner, and I had llama meat, which I would say tasted good. Puno was another delightful Inka town with its charming old houses, cobblestone streets, and hospitable tour guides. It was interesting to hear that the local soccer team always wins when the games are played in Puno because other teams were not trained to play at an altitude of twelve thousand feet.

Early in the morning, we had the traditional coca tea before we left for our tour. A double-decker bus transported us to a small harbor where a speed boat took us across Lake Titicaca, the highest navigable lake in the world, bordering with Bolivia. Our destination was the Uros Indian and Taquile Islands, the first one made from water reeds. We found out that there were forty big floating islands on the lake where people lived in harmony and strictly followed their customs and traditions. It was interesting to meet the people on the floating Uros Island, with faces withered from the wind and the sun. Most of them were young; we were told that because of the harsh climate conditions, people on these islands did not live past sixty years of age. They were properly dressed, as women had pretty, colorful dresses, and the children looked adorable in their festive outfits. After a brief cultural presentation, a girl took Mitt and I to show us the inside of their hut. The place was neat and clean, and the family slept on the ground with woolen blankets for covers. We learned that knitting was the most important part of their culture. What was surprising was that gender roles seemed to be reversed as to what we are accustomed to do in our lives. The boys, from an early age, had to learn how to knit, and that was their job as they grew older, while the girls did all the remaining work of farming, tending to the sheep, dying the wool, weaving, and spinning. The boys' knitting was serious as they had to learn this skill to get married. There were about two thousand inhabitants on the island, and they were all interrelated by blood or marriage. Their rules were simple: they had to live in peace and harmony, and anyone who disturbed it by improper behavior was expelled from the island. Then we had a tour on a boat that had an unusual decorative part in the front with a seat for two. We left the floating island, waving goodbye to these nice people, and they all waved back with big smiles. This was an exceptional scene of parting with people who had so much courage and great stamina to survive in such harsh conditions. It was the simplicity and beauty of life on this island which is a reminder of what is the most important thing in life, and that is to live in peace and harmony. There was another treat waiting for us on Taquile Island, which we were told is on a firm land. The scenery of the lake was gorgeous, tucked in the Andes Mountains that had different plants, such as the famous totora reed used for boat building, food, medicine, and bartering. We had to climb up a steep path to reach a place where a family had organized for us a lunch and dance performance event. However, as soon as I started to climb up the hill alongside the lake, I felt a pounding headache that is impossible to describe. I knew I was getting altitude sickness, but I did not want to give up and kept walking until we reached the place with a table set for lunch and meals ready to be served. It all looked delicious, but I couldn't taste a bite. However, I did get to enjoy the dances of the family. Then we climbed further up to a spot where they held their spiritual and festive activities. It was a spectacular view of pre-Inca ruins, terraced agricultural hills, and the mountains in the background.

Back on the boat I felt like passing out, and the captain gave me an oxygen mask, which helped me to a certain extent to reach town and find the first pharmacy in sight. The pharmacist knew exactly what to give me, and after a good night's rest I was ready for our next adventure in the tropical orchid capital of the world, Ecuador.

We arrived in Quito after midnight, which did not leave us much time to rest as our scheduled tour was at eight in the morning. The hotel was perfect; it was modern and very comfortable, so I could recover from the long trips and be on time for the tour.

Quito is an ancient Inca city, high in the Andean foothills with an altitude of 9,350 feet. I was eager to see the 16th and 17th centuries buildings of colonial times, the equator museum, and taste their food, which I heard is delicious.

Our guide was punctual and arrived at the scheduled time in the morning. He took us on a bus from the hotel to Guapulo Mirador, from where the views of the city at 9,300 feet are incredible. We passed by the Culture Center and the Legislative Palace in the historic part, where we stopped to view a very artistic mural art of the history of Ecuador. After Gran Columbia Avenue we reached the Basilica Catholic Church, which had the appearance of a cathedral, with its outside detailed architecture and beauty. We proceeded up a hill and soon reached El Mirador, a place that offered an extremely beautiful view of different parts of the entire city, like the upscale suburb of Cumbaya, the colonial part of town, as well as the Volcan Cayambe. The statue of Francisco was a figure of a Spaniard who looked down to the valley as a reminder of his first trip from Quito to the Atlantic.

The walk in the city's colonial streets was spectacular. We reached the independence plaza with a statue that commemorates the country's independence and those who fought for it. Around the plaza were magnificent government buildings, palaces, the historic Plaza Grande Hotel, and a majestic cathedral. I stood motionless for a while, trying to capture the magnificence of the place. I know all Latin American cities have plazas with a cathedral and government buildings around it, but there was something different about this place, as it seemed more European compared to the plazas in Peru. There were fountains, monuments, and statues that gave it a European look.

The tour continued to the attractive Sagrario and San Francisco churches. Both had an extremely glamourous architectural design. The San Francisco church was distinguishable with its two white towers by the main building. But it was Panecillo Miradora that I looked so much forward to seeing, with its phenomenal sites of old and new Quito. The tour followed its route to a beautiful park with flowers where a monument called La Mitad del

Mundo divided the Northern from the Southern Hemisphere. This was the place that I wanted to step foot on since I was a child, the Equator. I could feel my heartbeat when the guide told us the story about the monument that was built in the XVII century and how a French Expedition defined the equator line. Additional excitement was the visit to the Ethnographic Museum, which was accessible by elevator. Once on the top we passed pavilions that represented the countries that had expeditions to determine the location of the Equator. This was the first site for the location of the Equator, which was not exact because of lack of proper tools. The second place, which is a museum in a park, was extremely appealing. Here we walked on a line that marked the exact location of the Equator and staggered and swayed to the left and right as we felt forces that pulled us to the one and the other side. Here we watched an egg balanced on the tip of a nail. There was a sign showing zero latitude with a statue of an indigenous person from Ecuador, and at other decorative areas we saw statues of Inca images representing Ecuadorian daily life, as well as the different tribes and replicas of typical houses. At one pavilion they had bottles with sculpted people's heads, which was spooky. It was a reminder of the past when the indigenous people in this region performed such ceremonies in the past. One of the guys at the booth told us that his grandfather was involved in such rituals.

This visit to the Equator in Quito was priceless as no textbook can describe the excitement that I felt by stepping foot there.

The day continued to be full of exciting emotions, as, in the afternoon, a driver met us at the hotel and drove us to a resort in the Amazon Jungle. The trip was exhilarating, with the road twisting and turning among gorgeous mountainous sights, with hills of tropical vegetation and at the same time peaks covered with snow.

The complex of Jardin Aleman Lodge was an exceptional resort in the jungle. We entered a very well-kept and manicured park with tropical vegetation, greenery, trees and reached an outdoor restaurant that offered an amazing view of the jungle. As the evening approached, the birds started to make loud and unusual sounds. The host met us, and we were served a delicious three-course meal, after which we were taken to our house in the woods. The rooms were on the second floor with a living room, bedroom, and bathroom. There were ceiling fans and no air conditioner, which reminded me of the old days in Europe. The furniture was basic, a sofa and coffee table, two single beds, small side tables, and a closet. I smiled as I really liked this rustic lifestyle. We were the only guests at the resort and received a special treatment. The tours they had planned for us were extraordinary. The first day we went on a boat ride down the rivers Misahualli and Napo. We reached an indigenous settlement, at which we were treated with an indigenous dance performance while little monkeys jumped around. Then we took a walk in the forest, which was an adventure as we learned from the guide about different medicinal plants and the story of the trees which move towards the sun. The mere fact of being in the Amazon jungle and then learning about the flora and fauna was an extraordinary experience. The guide explained that one of the plants had hallucinogenic effects. He shared that he used the plant and had an amazing trip but that was because of his Indian culture, whereas tourists who experimented with it had a very bad time.

On the second day our guide handed us big rubber boots, and we set off on a trip through the jungle that was even more exciting than the first one as we had to pass through narrow areas surrounded by high rocks with bushes and jungle vegetation. It was hot, and sweat dripped down my face, but I felt energetic and energized. After a delicious lunch back at the Lodge, we were taken on another hike along the Misahuali River to visit the village Pununo. We crossed a suspended bridge and entered the Indian Community of Alto Pununo. The indigenous Ecuadorians were very friendly and waved as we walked by their homes. We backtracked to the resort, and on the way, I enjoyed the tropical jungle vegetation while listening to the stories of the guides.

During our stay we were entertained at the restaurant by the parrots Becky and Pedro, names that Mitt chose for them. They flew in every time we had a meal, landed on the back of a chair that was nearby, and patiently waited to be offered food. That added to the picturesque scenery of jungle life around us and became an everyday welcome sight.

Leaving Quito's airport and reminiscing on my experiences in Ecuador, I recommend visiting this amazing country on the Equator, a place so rich in folklore, history, and with breathtaking scenery.

PANAMA

I heard from a neighbor who visited Panama on a business trip about the splendor of this country and was curious to see this land of paradise, with splendid white sand beaches, a mysterious jungle, and the man-made wonder of the world, the Panama Canal.

It was late in the evening when we arrived in Panama City. The Latin Escapes tour representative met us at the airport and drove us to our hotel, Holiday Inn, located at a walking distance from the Panama Canal lock, which we were scheduled to see in the morning.

Our first visit was to Miraflores Lock, one of the three locks named after a small manmade lake, Miraflores, of the Panama Canal, connecting it to Pedro Miquel Locks. It was a sight to see with your own eyes to fully appreciate it. The great body of water twisted across the tropics, with enormous freighters perfectly lined up to cross the canal. The guide explained that there were three locks, and the Miraflores was the biggest, with a height compared to that of a six-story building. I immediately climbed on the observation decks to get a better view of the entire area. Huge freighters waited to cross the canal, and the one that was right in front my eyes almost touched both of its sides. They said that usually about forty freighters pass the canal daily after two to three days of a wait. We were lucky to observe a freighter cross the canal at the time when the ship was lowered to sea level. Then we peeked at the museum to learn the entire process of crossing the canal. The guide also told us the story about the efforts to build the canal, first by the French, and then by the Americans. The French operation failed because working conditions were disastrous. The use of opium was what kept the workers digging, and many of them died of yellow fever and malaria. The American project was successful because they addressed the issue of disease control. They also introduced a very innovative concept of creating locks as opposed to the French approach, which was to build a canal at sea level.

This morning we also visited the other two locks, San Pedro Miquel and Gatun, the latter being the largest with three chambers. Incredible sights of man-built canals of such greatness and importance are a must see in a person's life.

Our second stop was at the ruins of Panama Viejo, the oldest Spanish settlement on the Pacific. The city boomed in the past with trade, and ships traveled to Spain transporting gold and silver. This caught the eye of pirates and the Welsh Henry Morgan, who was a famous pirate and whose name is now on the rum bottles. They destroyed the city in the 1600s. The city is currently a UNESCO site. It is a historical gem with its cathedral viewing tower and ruins of buildings connected by paths.

Our driver took us next to the charming colonial settlement Casco Viejo, where Captain Morgan's crew settled and established a very attractive place with old colorful homes and cobblestone streets. It was so hot that I remember how refreshing was the bottle of beer we shared before continuing to one of the Amador Islands. The island was charming with its tropical vegetation, and we stopped to relax and enjoy the view of the water with its changing blue colors. We decided to walk the six kilometers causeway to Panama City, where people biked and exercised alongside the ocean. Panama City looked so spectacular in the distance with its skyscrapers and newer buildings. There was an area on our way that looked somewhat questionable, and a guy with a car stopped to give us a ride to where it was safe for tourists. That was a very unexpected gesture, and we both appreciated the friendliness of this stranger. It was dark when we arrived in the city. We entered a mall and stopped at a fast-food court where we had a delicious Latin American dish. I was so tired that I looked at Mitt and told him that the mattress store across looked so attractive, at which he laughed. I was in no condition to walk more, so we took a cab to the hotel.

Early in the morning I jumped out of bed, as I knew that we were going to the Gamboa Rainforest Reserve in the jungle, and that was enough of an incentive to make me forget how tired I was the previous night. The ride to the resort was fabulous through tropical forests and luxuriant vegetation, with birds making loud sounds in the trees. The hotel was amazing, with an outdoor lobby overlooking swimming pools in the back. Further in the distance were green meadows, trees, bushes, and the Chagres River. And our room had the same incredible tropical scenery. There was a hammock on the terrace, which I immediately hopped on with a glass of fresh fruit pina colada in my hand. *This is life*, I thought to myself.

When we travel, I always need to know about the animals in the area, and the receptionist told me that there were jaguars, tapirs, sloths, anteaters, but assured us that jaguars do not roam in the tourist places. I could see tapirs and anteaters from the terrace. And sloths were hanging on the trees when we took a very exhilarating canoe trip on Chagres River with tropical forests on both sides. What was also memorable was the resort's aerial tram tour, which offered the most panoramic views of the forest with breathtaking flora, followed by a visit to a butterfly farm where I saw the most beautiful blue butterflies.

Later in the day it was time to jump in the pool and unwind after a magnificent, unforgettable day in the Panama's jungle.

We were supposed to see Colon, but the tour company in Panama decided to change it to a historic attraction, Fort San Lorenzo. A young man picked us up in the morning and drove us to the Atlantic side of the country. Fort San Lorenzo, as the name suggests, has its walls and watch tower used by the Spaniards to detect pirates. We walked by the walls, where there were canons, and ruins and enjoyed the beautiful view of River Chagres that flows into the bay. We also visited an old Catholic church with a Black Jesus where the local villagers prayed and had services. On the way back we stopped for lunch in a very folkloric decorated in Panamanian-style restaurant.

The last place that we visited in Panama was a luxurious beach resort on the Pacific Ocean with a white sandy beach. We checked in the hotel and immediately headed out. Mitt bought a cigar, and we sat in lounge chairs by the pool when he turned to me and said that he had not felt relaxed like that in quite a while. After days of heaven in the sun, we headed back to Texas, our home now.

CHAPTER 22
Maldives—Heaven On Earth

"See Venice and die" is not an accurate saying anymore, since there are so many magnificent, picturesque, breathtaking places on earth, and the islands of the Maldives are one of them. Our flight from Bulgaria to Male was shorter than what it would have been if we traveled from the States. We had a long layover in Doha, Qatar, and the travel agency that we used in Sofia offered a sightseeing tour. I have to say that the trip was very well organized with good directions and instructions for tickets and meeting places. We took a bus to the Arabian city that I was so curious to see. We live in Texas, and I should be used to heat, but the 105-degree temperature late in the evening and without any wind was a little too much even for a Texan. I wore a scarf and covered my arms to fit in the Muslim culture, which made me feel even more uncomfortable. Nonetheless I enjoyed all the sights on this tour. Our first stop was across the water of Doha's Corniche, with a magnificent view of Doha's skyline at night, which was illuminated with skyscrapers in blue, red, orange, green, and purple colors. Then we stopped at a mosque and the opera house at Katara Cultural village, which was a popular place for cultural events and recreation. There was a mall and buildings of striking and artistic modern architecture. We continued our tour and viewed from the bus the museum of Islamic art and the national museum of Qatar. Both buildings were amazing of unique modern architecture but very distinct from each other. The National Museum reminded me of the opera house in Sidney with its unusual design, and the museum of Islamic art resembled a luxurious hotel. At Souq Waqii Market, we had time to explore and get acquainted with local night life. I was surprised to see that it was different from the souks of Dubai or Istanbul. We walked down a street with cafes, restaurants, and shops. The guide told us that the fire in 2003 destroyed most of the market, and that was the reason for its new look. We had an hour of free time to venture on our own. There were people at the outside cafes, and I wondered how they seemed not to be bothered by the heat. We knew that we had to find a place with air conditioning. The café we walked in was not a tourist spot as only locals sat at the tables. I knew what I wanted, freshly baked flatbread, falafel, and sweet dumplings that looked like donuts. A quick drive back to the airport and we were on our way to our destination, the Maldives.

I have saved the best for last, a place of heaven on earth, with numerous coral islands of different shapes in plush tropical vegetation, with powder sand beaches surrounded by the most beautiful multicolored blue waters of the Indian Ocean. We circled over Male, the capital, and I could not help but admire the buildings of different colors with red-tile roofs by the splendid water. When we landed, we were instructed to head to an airport with seaplanes. That was our second time flying out of such an airport with seaplanes parked in the water. We were about to fly to Kuredu Island and were just as excited as when a couple of summers ago we traveled to Velidhu, a smaller island. Kuredu Island had its own seaplanes, which were bigger, and the transfer was faster. I nestled myself by the window and glued my face to the glass not to miss any of the beautiful scenery below of scattered small islands of unique shape and form. The plane flew low, and I could make out even the people on the beaches, and the colors of the corals. We landed in the water by the pier and were welcomed by a local singing and dancing group. Check-in was expedited, and a golf cart took us to our beach house. I felt like I was in paradise when I walked out on the beach and stepped on the powder-like white sand with tropical plants and palm trees around. The front porch had a daybed and a dining room set. There were a couple of lounge chairs on the beach between palm trees. It was a luxurious villa with an outdoor enclosed bathroom in the back that was decorated with plants and flowers. Ahh, life on the beach. We dropped off our luggage in the room and went for a walk to discover what the place had to offer. There were houses on stilts in the water, and we headed towards them. We wanted to see if we could spot fish as we did at Velidhu Island, where there was an abundance of the most beautiful colorful fish I had ever seen by the pier. What we saw were a couple of coral sharks that swam next to each other. Further on the beach was a sandy path that went straight into the sea, a very unusual sight that I painted once I returned home. We came across a restaurant with a beautiful view from a terrace on the water and had a refreshing drink. Feeling refreshed we continued our walk and came across a soccer field, a golf course, and tennis courts. Following the path, we reached a beach restaurant and three other very attractive restaurants with exclusive menus, as well as beach bars by the reception. There were water villas, a spa, three pools, a fitness scenter, water sports, and bikes. It was such an invigorating atmosphere that I felt like dancing. It took two hours to walk all over the island, which is more than at Velidhu, where it took only half an hour. We stopped at a travel agency by the reception and booked sunset and snorkeling boat tours. The sunset cruise was spectacular, with beautiful sunrays of orange and gold colors dancing on the water, and to make the scene even more perfect, we saw dolphins.

The reef safari snorkeling was an amazing and extremely thrilling experience. We were taken to two reefs, and I couldn't wait to jump in the water as soon as we stopped. I was at once surrounded by colorful fish of all kinds and sizes. I loved the blue ones with yellow stripes, and the multicolor bigger fish with a predominant blue color, but also green, pink, and orange. I was in complete bliss. Then I decided to check out the deep part close to the reef where the water was dark blue. I looked down and spotted a shadow of a stingray coming straight at me. My heart jumped, and I cleared out of this place as fast as I could.

That evening we attended a Maldives cultural show with a documentary film about the history of the islands. There was an art presentation with paintings from local artists and Maldives dancing, which I was so happy to join in.

The two weeks flew by fast. Life on the beach was like a dream. Waking up with the morning sunrise to greet the first sunrays on the water and walking out the door right on the beach was a joyous experience beyond description. Our days were full of delightful activities. We swam and snorkeled by the beach, took long walks, and enjoyed the delicious local cuisine. One day I had a massage which I cannot forget because lying face down, I could watch fish through a glass floor.

We spent the evenings by the bar on the pier and watched stingrays and sharks give spectacular shows under the lit-up area over the water. What I loved the most about both islands was the fact that I walked everywhere barefoot and snorkeled every day by the pier at Velidhu and at the beach of Kuredu amidst the most beautiful and colorful fish I had seen on earth.

SUMMARY: PART TWO

I hope you enjoyed the chapters of my travel around the world and received sufficient information and understanding of what traveling means and how it affects our health. This is not an inclusive list of countries that I visited, as some of my travels are described in my debut book and others I took while writing this book.

In conclusion, after sharing most of my travel experiences, I would like to capture some of the major benefits from them.

Travel is the only way to engage all parts of your body and your mind and to be active during the entire time that you are awake. The moment you wake up in a strange new place, your mind is focused on activities for the day. If you are going on a tour, you will immediately think about its name, what you are going to see, what and where is the meeting place, what you need to pack and take with you, where you are going to have your first sip of coffee. If you decide to explore a place on your own, you need to select the most attractive and recommended places to visit, you need to find out what times are opening and closing hours for museums or other attractions, what is the cost for entering and attending events, and what are necessary items to carry with you; do not forget your camera or phone for taking photos. In both situations you need to be organized so you can have a stress-free and pleasant experience. Most important is to know the foreign currency exchange rate and have enough cash on you as well as a credit card. In some countries, as in China, you need to carry a passport to enter sightseeing locations, and in others you might need to have some form of identification. An independent traveler has more challenges, such as organizing modes of transportation, booking of hotels, sightseeing tours arrangements, etc.

First, we are going to examine the benefits of performing physical activities while traveling. From the moment you wake up to bedtime, you are in constant movement. You are walking, hiking, swimming, snorkeling, biking and more, depending on the activities you choose for the day. Whether you are doing a city tour, visiting museums, and shopping, hopping on funiculars or boats, or climbing a hill to view a beautiful panorama of the city or the countryside, you are in constant movement that requires the use of all your body muscles and senses.

The benefits do not stop here. Whether on a tour or on your own, you constantly learn, view, listen, touch, examine, inhale, taste, and admire presentations that the world reveals to you. When you are at archeological sites and in old cities, you learn about history from ancient times to today, and the visual aspect of being at those locations contributes to an experience that history books cannot replace.

You learn geography in a way that can never be presented in a geography lesson. Whether you are in the jungle, on top of a mountain, at the beach or in the city, you will always remember the names, the views, and the smells of those places that impressed you so much.

Images and names of plants and animals will remain with you forever as you associate them with the natural habitat of the place you visited.

You will get a better perspective of the world's economy when you visit countries on different continents. Lessons in economics on location are invaluable for understanding and being able to make a comparison between the economy of a country we visit with the one we live in.

Attending cultural events and performances of music, dancing, and acting, interacting with local people and learning about their lifestyle, tasting food with ingredients of vegetables and spices that we are not familiar with are all precious memories with a significant impact on our mental health.

Meeting people, making friends, and forming long-lasting relationships contributes as well to our mental stability. When we interact with people of different upbringings, social standings, and education, we enrich our understanding about the world and the importance of valuable life issues. Contact with people around the globe permits us to reevaluate our thinking and understanding of all aspects of life. There is a saying that in one place people live to work, whereas in another they work to live. Travel teaches the value of memories and beauty as opposed to that of material objects.

In summary, I would like to say that life is a journey, and that we are the ones who define its course.

CONCLUSION

We have one life to live, and it is our choice of how to live it. Living a happy and healthy life is a state of mind as we have the power and ability to determine how to spend our time. We are the ones in control of how to schedule and spend our daily activities by setting and achieving goals. In reference to sustaining a healthy body and mind, we create a routine or a habit which promotes healthy living. What is important is that we choose activities and set goals that we love to do and are passionate about. I encourage my readers to explore all possibilities for engaging in beneficial practices to discover what suits them best. The easiest ways to be active are to walk, jog, or run, and from there on you may add any of the practices that I suggest or the ones that you select on your own.

This book provides guidelines with examples of my physical and mental exercises, nutrition, and activities to maintain my health, looks, and spirits as well as the benefits that I derive from them. It also calls our attention to treat our body and mind with respect, paying attention to what is required to sustain a good physical and mental condition. It teaches you how to pace yourself and listen to your body to avoid injuries, as you do not have to imitate other people. Enjoy practices that suit you best and are most appealing to you. Feel every part of your body when you move, breathe, and absorb the sunrays or listen to the whisper of the trees, the chirping of the birds, or the roaring of the sea when by water. Admire every moment that nature gifts you with its paintings of glamourous colors and shapes of clouds in the sky, of changing green colors of leaves on the trees, bushes, and shrubs in the forest; the variety of kinds and colors of flowers; and the beautiful shades of blue colors of the seas. This is the beginning of your journey to a happy and self-fulfilled life.

What is essential for this book is that it provides a balanced approach to physical and mental activities. My daily schedule is a mix of selected activities from studying Chinese to walking, playing the piano, biking, writing, swimming, cooking, and others based on availability and season. I find it necessary that to be productive I need to alternate physical and mental activities. Such an approach assists me to be successful at what I plan to accomplish, which in turn gives me satisfaction and pleasure. For those who spend their days in offices, it is beneficial to engage in physical exercises before or after work, and for blue collar workers, it is preferable to have mental exercises, such as reading, answering trivia questions, or solving crossword puzzles. I am not a morning person, so, when I worked, I visited the gym, walked, or rode a bike in the evening. It is important to note that the list of suggested exercises and foods is not all inclusive and can be adjusted for each person's unique background, being Asian-Pacific, African, or Indian. I am of European background, and most of the food and my exercises are based on my origin, but I also added new activities and nutrition from my travel experiences.

The book also addresses the importance of being relaxed and in the proper state of mind to achieve a well-balanced and healthy life. Our relationships with family, friends, and social interactions are essential for a life in peace and tranquility. Keeping in contact with people who support us, understand us, and love us is just as important as the air we breathe.

We as human beings need to pursue our dreams and goals at all ages. It is never too late to pick up an instrument, paint, dance, or sing. I am living proof of that as I picked up playing the piano and painting after retirement. And the same is true for physical practices as I overcame my anxiety of going underwater, and snorkeling became my preferred water sport. Be patient, recognize and praise yourself for each advancement and achievement you make in whatever you do. It takes hours, days, months, and years of practice and dedication to improve in your activity, so just sit back and enjoy the process.

The book also provides an exclusive study of benefits derived from travel. The purpose of the chapters for travel around the world is to demonstrate the all-encompassing advantage gained from visiting foreign lands and places. The variety of programs and activities keep the mind and body engaged from early morning till dusk. For example, in a visit to Macho Picchu, I learned all about Peruvian history and culture, the origin of the complex, its abandonment and subsequent discovery. I also climbed steps up and down and walked quite a bit to view all the places described and pointed out by the tour guide. The added privilege was to admire such a majestic place surrounded by mountains with llamas peeking from behind the hill.

Starting with an organized tour by a travel agency is a safe and comforting approach to venture into the unknown. There are chapters in the book about trips to South America organized by Latin Escapes travel agency. We used travel agencies in Bulgaria to book trips to Israel and the Maldives, which took care of arrangements for our flights, transfers, and stay at all-inclusive hotels. Travel on cruise ships as described by Oceania, Star Clippers and Royal Caribbean cruise lines to countries in Africa, Asia, and Europe is also stress-free, as all land excursions and activities on board are organized by the destination desks and the cruise director. Whether on a cruise ship or a trip booked by a travel agency, you are guaranteed a set itinerary of sightseeing, exploration, and activities. When you gain more confidence, you can start organizing your own trips on the internet, booking your own flights, hotels, and researching places to visit. Such experience is described in the book in chapters describing the use of Eurail to travel around Europe and fast trains in France and Spain. The Eurail trip is for an adventurer at heart and requires good organizational and planning skills.

Whatever activity and way of life you choose depends entirely on you. It is our thoughts and hearts which guide us how to act and what to pursue. The book is an invitation to engage in activities which promote a healthy, happy life and a reminder to be true to yourself. What is important is to keep moving and to follow your dreams and goals.

APPENDIX
Bulgarian Traditional Recipes

TARATOR

A refreshing summer cold soup. The benefits of this dish are enormous. Apart from being very tasty and thirst-quenching, it has ingredients with a health significance. Cucumber has antioxidants; its high-water content helps with hydration. I use Bulgarian yogurt, but Greek or any other plain yogurt will be fine. Bulgarian yogurt has lactobacillus—a bacteria supporting the immune system, which as a probiotic product is extremely healthy; garlic and walnuts also boost the immune system; walnuts are rich in antioxidants.

Ingredients

One cucumber

2 cups non-fat Bulgarian or Greek yoghurt

4 crushed walnuts

Dill—chopped.

A spoonful of olive oil

A pinch of salt

Crushed garlic

Grate the cucumber, stir in the yoghurt, the walnuts, the dill, garlic, oil, and salt. Add water for density as you prefer. Stir and serve in soup bowls. Eat with pogacha bread.

Antonina Duridanova

POGACHA bread

Benefits from pogacha are that it is all natural and extremely tasty. Milk has calcium, eggs provide quality protein and have vitamin D; butter has also vitamin D.

Ingredients
5 cups all-purpose flour
1 cup of milk
1 egg
1 active dry yeast
5 tbs. melted butter
¼ vegetable oil
Half a teaspoon salt and half a teaspoon sugar
1 cup sour cream

Heat the milk, add the melted butter, and let cool off for 15 min. Add yeast, sugar, salt, and stir to mix well and have it dissolved. Let it rise – 15 min.

Have the flour in a bowl and make a hole in the middle; pour in it the milk and butter mixture, a well beaten egg, the oil, the sour cream (sour cream can be substituted with grated cheese of your choice). Knead the mixture until elastic, then cover and let rise in a warm place (I usually use the oven) for about an hour.

Place the dough on a lightly covered surface with flour, divide in desired forms, then transfer to a greased bowl, flipping to grease on both sides. Bake at 335 F for about an hour. Pogacha can be served with other dishes—baked beans, vegetable, and meat dishes.

MISH-MASH

This is a meal which can be prepared for any time of the day. The Bulgarian mish mash is a dish of scrambled eggs with vegetables—chopped peppers, tomatoes, onion, parsley, feta cheese, and sweet paprika. Benefits from this dish are great—tomatoes are rich in vitamin C and potassium, onions contain antioxidants, and sweet paprika has antioxidant properties; for other ingredients, refer to summer salad recipe.

Fry in olive oil the peppers, onions, and tomatoes until water evaporates. Stir in eggs and mix until they are well mixed with the vegetables and cooked (do not overcook). Sprinkle paprika and stir, sprinkle chopped parsley and serve with pogacha.

STUFFED PEPPERS, EGGPLANT, TOMATOES, ZUCCHINI
(You may combine or use any of the vegetables separately.)

Ingredients: 1 lb. ground meat (beef, bison, or veal), half a pound mild Italian sausage or Spanish chorizo, one chopped onion, one sliced carrot, a cut stalk of celery, 5–6 mushrooms, 3–4 pieces of garlic, paprika, salt, turmeric powder, sweet pepper, oregano or summer savory, vegetable broth, one can crushed tomatoes or two tomatoes, olive oil, spaghetti sauce, one cup of basmati rice.

Bake eggplant and peppers (mixture of red, green, orange) in oven at 320 F until slightly soft (not fully baked); spoon out the middle of the eggplant and add to the meat mixture.

Meat mixture: Cook all other ingredients on the stove in a pan sprayed with olive oil and covered with a lid. Mix the meat so there are no chunks of it. Add salt, black pepper, sweet pepper, turmeric, oregano, mix well. Cook until the meat is brown and vegetables slightly soft. Cook rice in rice cooker, and when done, stir in the meat and vegetable mixture.

Arrange the peppers (sometimes I divide them in half), eggplants, tomatoes, and zucchini in a baking dish. Spoon the meat mixture inside the peppers (sometimes I cut them in half), eggplants, zucchini, tomatoes. Pour over vegetable broth to cover one third of the baking dish. Pour over spaghetti sauce evenly to cover all vegetables. Cover with a lid and bake at 390 F for 30 min. Turn off oven. Remove lid and let stay in oven 15–20 min. before serving.

SUMMER SALAD

Ingredients: Lettuce; tomatoes; cucumbers; hot pepper; pepperoncini; chopped green, red, and peppers; olives; red onion, or green onions; avocado; olives; parsley; vinegar; olive oil; feta cheese. The health benefits of this salad are tremendous. Lettuce has carotene; peppers, olives are rich in oxidants; avocado contains C, E, K vitamins, magnesium, potassium and more healthy attributes; parsley has vitamin K—found good for bone growth; feta cheese has more calcium than other cheeses—good for bone health.

Place diced tomatoes, cucumbers, cut peppers, chopped red onion or green onions, parsley in a salad bowl, arrange olives around the bowl. Prepare vinegar and oil dressing in a small bowl, add oregano, pour the dressing over the salad, and mix well; arrange avocado slices on top and sprinkle with lemon or lime. Grate feta cheese abundantly over the salad. Arrange olives around the bowl. Enjoy.

You may replace tomatoes with watermelon cubes.

BULGARIAN VEAL PAPRIKASH

Ingredients: 4–5 red peppers, onion, garlic, sweet pepper, one pound veal or chicken, olive oil, salt, black pepper, sweet paprika, bay leaf, parsley, vegetable broth, one tablespoon flour.

Health benefits—Black pepper has antioxidants; bay leaf has vitamins A, B6 and C, which support the immune system; veal meat has vitamins B12 and D, iron; and chicken has nutrients like protein, niacin, phosphorus; other ingredients described in mish mash and tarator recipes.

Simmer on stove top cubes of meat, sliced peppers, chopped onion, and garlic. Cook until the meat and vegetables are tender, sprinkle a tablespoon of paprika, stir and cook for a minute, add vegetable broth, bay leaf, salt, and black pepper. Cook another 5-10 min. For thicker soup, pour with a ladle a cup of the hot broth from the paprikas in a dish, add a tablespoon of flour, mix well to break up any lumps, then return to the pot. Mix and cook for a couple of minutes. Sprinkle with parsley and serve. Serve with mashed potatoes or small potatoes sprinkled with sea salt and paprika and baked in a baking dish sprayed with olive oil and a tablespoon of vegetable broth. You can also serve it with white rice and quinoa.

GJUBECH – BULGARIAN DISH – BAKED MEAT WITH VEGETABLES

Ingredients: One pound veal, beef, or lamb meat; 1 lb. green beans, one eggplant, can of crushed tomatoes or 2 tomatoes, tomato paste, two peppers (green and red), one onion, 4 pieces of garlic, a can of peas (can be frozen), 3–4 potatoes, ½ lb. okra, summer savory (chubritsa—careful as in English they translate chubritsa as sharena sol, which is not the same) or oregano, 1 tbs. sweet paprika, 1 tbs. turmeric, a pinch of black pepper, ½ tbs. cumin, sea salt, ½ tbs. coriander, 2 tbs. olive oil.

Benefits—This dish is full of nutrients; some ingredients described in other recipes from above; summer savory is loaded with nutrients—calcium, iron, vitamin B6, magnesium, protein, fiber; peas; okra contain antioxidants; cumin has antioxidants; coriander has vitamin A, turmeric has curcumin, known for its anti-inflammatory properties; eggplant is rich in fiber and antioxidants; potatoes contain vitamin C and potassium.

Best cooked in a clay pot, but a baking pot like Le Creuset with a lid can also be used.

Marinate meat in a bowl mixed with paprika, salt, black pepper, a pinch of coriander, cumin and turmeric, spoon of olive oil, crushed garlic, and oregano or summer savory.

Clean and cut the peppers, onion, potatoes, okra, green beans, eggplant (in cubes). Mix salt, pepper, paprika, and oregano or chubritsa with the vegetables.

Layer the pot first with the marinated meat, then the vegetables without the potatoes. Cover with a cup of vegetable broth. Combine the tomato paste, tomatoes, or crushed tomatoes, oregano, and pour over the vegetables.

Cover the pot and bake at 410 F for 30 min. Add the potatoes cut in a shape you prefer and return to oven uncovered for another 30 min., or when potatoes are golden; add frozen peas. Let stay in warm oven for another 10 min. Sprinkle with parsley and serve.

MUSSAKA – BULGARIAN AND GREEK DISH

Bulgarians make this dish with potatoes, and Greeks with eggplant.
I will show the recipe with eggplant and potatoes.

Ingredients: 1 lb. ground meat (beef, bison, or veal), half a pound mild Italian sausage or Spanish chorizo, one chopped onion, one sliced carrot, a stalk of celery, 5–6 mushrooms, two tomatoes or a can of crushed tomatoes, 3–4 pieces of garlic, paprika, salt, turmeric powder, sweet pepper, oregano or summer savory, vegetable broth, olive oil, 4–5 potatoes or 2 eggplants.

Benefits—Most ingredients discussed in gjuvech recipe: carrots have vitamin A and beta carotene; celery has numerous vitamins, among them potassium and calcium; mushrooms are a source of fiber, antioxidants, and protein.

In a pan, cook the meat with the vegetables and spices until meat is browned and vegetables are soft. Boil potatoes, and when cooked, but not completely as for mashed potatoes, chop them into small squares; mix with the rest of the ingredients and cover evenly with bechamel sauce. If using eggplant, slice the eggplants horizontally, cook on very low temperature to soften. Layer in the baking pot—first meat mixture, then slices of eggplant, pour bechamel sauce evenly to cover generously the entire top layer.

Bake at 410F for 30 min., or when top layer becomes golden.

Bechamel sauce recipes are available on the internet.

BANITSA

The most well-known Bulgarian dish served anytime, but mostly mornings with a side dish of yogurt. It is a very nutritional all-natural breakfast or anytime snack.

You can use ready-made dough, or you can make your own dough, which is not complicated; it just takes practice as you need to roll it into very thin sheets. This recipe is with ready-made dough.

Ingredients: One package of ready-made dough, ¼ cup melted butter, half container of yogurt, olive oil, feta cheese, package of ricotta cheese, two eggs.

Crumble the feta cheese, add the ricotta, the eggs (save the yoke of one), spoonful of olive oil (you can add spinach or cooked leek if you prefer).

Melt the butter and mix with yogurt.

On a baking dish sprayed with olive oil, start layering the sheets—three sheets, 2 sheets with spread of butter and yogurt mixture, third sheet with evenly spread cheese mixture. Spread evenly on the top sheet a layer of butter, yogurt, and egg yolk mixture.

Bake at 325 F for half an hour or until golden color.

Banitsa has many variations of preparing and cooking; some may be layered with yellow cheese,*kashkaval*, or ham.

Antonina Duridanova

PUMPKIN BANITSA

For dessert I am offering you Pumpkin Banitsa—
my father's favorite dessert.

Ingredients: Ready-made dough, grated pumpkin (one and a half pounds), olive oil, crushed walnuts, cinnamon, unsalted butter (half a stick).

Mix the grated pumpkin with the cinnamon and walnuts.

Layer the sheets of dough and spray two with olive oil, while spreading the pumpkin mixture entirely on the third sheet. Put small pieces of butter on the last sheet at the corners, the sides, and some in the middle.

Bake at 325 F for half an hour, or when the top layer has golden color.

KEBAPCHETA ON GRILL

Ingredients
I kg. of ground meat (70/30 pork/beef)
Cumin – 1 teaspoon
Salt – 1–2 teaspoons
Black pepper – ground, 1–2 teaspoons
Carbonated water or beer – 600 ml.

Benefits – Ground beef is a good source of energy, providing several vitamin Bs and protein. Ground pork has vitamins B and 12, protein, zinc, and iron. The recipe's healthy spices are addressed above.

Mix well all ingredients with half the water or beer.

Let it stay for 1 hr. or more.

Add the remaining water, or beer, and mix well again.

Form elongated kebapcheta 10–14 cm. long and diameter up to 3 cm.

Grill on a very hot grill, turning over in 5 min.

Serve hot with fried potatoes, salad, and a choice of grilled vegetables (peppers, zucchini, corn).

Printed in the USA
CPSIA information can be obtained
at www.ICGtesting.com
LVHW020458020524
778878LV00013B/470